Praise for *Wolves,*

Wolves, Gardens, and Chocolate is chock-full of holistic health wisdom. It's a winner.
Christiane Northrup, MD, OB/GYN physician and author of the *New York Times* best-sellers *Goddesses Never Age: The Secret Prescription for Radiance, Vitality, and Wellbeing*; *Women's Bodies, Women's Wisdom*; and *The Wisdom of Menopause*

Doctors are trained to treat the result and not the cause. However, people are not mechanical objects and need to be treated in a holistic way which integrates mind, body, and spirit. *Wolves, Gardens, and Chocolate* offers us guidance and insight into this integrated pattern of self care and medical care. We all need coaching in our lives when we encounter problems, and Dr. Arrondo's wisdom can become your guide to better health and life.
Bernie Siegel, MD, author of *Love, Medicine & Miracles* and *The Art of Healing*; Assistant Clinical Professor of General and Pediatric Surgery, Yale University, retired.

Dr. Arrondo's book is a fantastic book for anyone seeking effective strategies to improve their health.
Datis Kharrazian, DHSc, DC, MS, FAACP, DACBN, DABCN, DIBAK, CNS, research fellow at Harvard Medical School and the Department of Neurology at Massachusetts General Hospital. Associate Clinical Professor, Loma Linda University School of Medicine, author of *Why Do I Still Have Thyroid Symptoms When My Lab Tests Are Normal?* and *Why Isn't My Brain Working?*

Dr. Arrondo has given you the key to preventing disease and the foundation for recovering from the diseases of civilization!
C. Norman Shealy, MD, PhD, author of *Living Bliss* and *90 Days to Self-Health*

A wide-ranging discussion on well-being that offers plenty of food for thought and action. Overall, it's a valuable holistic-health roundup.
Kirkus Reviews

Wolves, Gardens, and Chocolate offers a gift to readers not found in most natural health books: an intriguing and expansive approach to healing that integrates the deepest levels of our lives. Dr. Arrondo has written an invaluable healing aid.
Gerald Roliz, CNC, author of *The Pharmaceutical Myth*

Dr. Arrondo's book will help you find the health, energy, and inspiration you have been looking for. In this detailed, referenced tome is a roadmap to health—from the theoretical to the practical, from the simple to the complex. It has hundreds of simple steps you can take to regain and maximize your health. A must read!
Dr. Brian Kelly, President, Life Chiropractic College–West

Dr. Arrondo provides a discerning and penetrating discussion of ourselves immersed in modern health-care delivery. The practice of health care is about evolution, and *Wolves, Gardens, and Chocolate* bestows much foundation knowledge to make improved choices in that evolution. *Wolves* is a good read for clinicians and consumers alike.
Steve Cohen, MD, PA-C, Associate Professor, Florida International University, Miami

A book that will be enjoyed by physicians and patients alike, *Wolves, Gardens, and Chocolate* addresses each concept and medical situation with great clarity. Dr. Arrondo illustrates through didactic analogies, as well as his valuable humanistic-clinical experience.
Susana Alcázar, MD, Director of Hans Selye Scientific Research Institute, A.C., Founder and Director of Herberto Alcázar Montenegro School of Gerontology, S.C.

In our "modern world" there is an urgent need to reassess how we think and act about health and wellness. *Wolves, Gardens, and Chocolate* is an excellent primer, providing the essential information you need to know about improving your health from a highly experienced clinician.
Kerry Bone, Director Research & Development—MediHerb; Adjunct Professor—School of Applied Clinical Nutrition, New York Chiropractic College

This is a journal, kept by a compassionate observationalist devoted to philosophy who intends to freely and openly draw from lessons he learned or heard of along the way of his journey. Everyone has their hand gently held as you follow along being nourished by fascinating stories that lead you to a better life without all that effort nearly everyone tells us we should take.
Gerald Paul Kozlowski, PhD, BCN, Board Certified Senior Fellow in Neurofeedback, Department of Clinical Psychology, Saybrook University

Dr. Arrondo has done a wonderful job in explaining and demonstrating how *every* system in our body is inseparable and must function seamlessly to maintain health. This book provides insight in how improving the function/wellness of one "dis-eased" system (imbalanced microbiomes in and on our bodies, negative internal monologues, inflammatory eating, etc.) can inflate the wellness/functioning of the whole body.
Paul D. Walton, BS, DC, CCSP, Professor, Life Chiropractic College West

I am excited to have such a book available to recommend to my patients. *Wolves, Gardens, and Chocolate* is a wonderful book about reestablishing and maintaining health in a post-millennial world.
Erich Goetzel, MD, MA, LAc

Dr. Arrondo aptly presents the readers practical advice on how to achieve healthier and happier lives by understanding and using these delicate physical, mental, and spiritual interconnections to our benefit. In a medical universe of increasingly subspecialized medical training, Dr. Arrondo's book reminds us of the importance of this holistic approach to modern medicine.
Michael C. Kuo, MD

Finally, a new, evidence-based approach to address the true causes of much pain and suffering. More importantly, a true patient-based approach. Thanks, Dr. Arrondo, for this evidence-based and patient-based attempt to educate the public about the powerful choices that they can make to determine their level of health, illness, and lifespan.
Edward Cremata, DC, RN, FRCP(US), Professor, Palmer College of Chiropractic West

Dr. Arrondo has written an excellent book that will help everyone learn how to better take care of their health. His well-researched book helps show the many connections between the different systems in our body and gives practical suggestions at the end of every chapter. Read this book and you will learn to think about your health in a more holistic way.
Richard Chen, MD, FAAFP, IFMCP

Dr. Arrondo explains that when we are out of alignment with our life's purpose or life is somehow out of balance, disease and dysfunction can result, often as a wake-up call to get our attention and move us to make the necessary life/lifestyle changes. He offers suggestions on how to make changes and to find answers when we discover ourselves with ill health that we cannot seem to turn around. I highly recommend this book as a guide to all who seek optimal health and healing.
Deanna M. Cherrone, MD

This is a wonderful explanation of the mind-body connection. Dr. Arrondo gives power back to the patient, teaching self-reliance and empowerment. Not that doctors are unimportant, but listening to our own body is just as important. Thank you for showing us all how much power we have over our own health.
Susan Rhodes, RN, MS, LMFT, PsyD

Dr. Arrondo has amalgamated science and his wisdom to help all of us navigate an ever more confusing world of "healthy choices." *Wolves, Gardens, and Chocolate* is a must-read for young and old. The information in this book can bring pragmatism and simplification to the complex subject of healthy living. Read, enjoy, and follow Dr. Arrondo on a journey toward optimal health.
Louis D'Amico, DC, BS Pharmacy, RPh

Many thanks for distilling such a vast body of research into this amazing roadmap to vitality. I have already recommended Dr. Arrondo's book to a number of patients. It has been such a wonderful synthesis of many of the elements that I work with patients on in clinic, and has helped to revitalize my approach to some of the conditions that I treat regularly.
Rain Delvin, EAMP, MAOM, LMP

Dr. Arrondo presents a science-based approach to health care that engages and empowers the patient who is seeking to learn about their health and improve their health. The rich scientific information is artfully and skillfully interwoven with traditional, cultural, culinary, and healing practices dating back to antiquity. The information flows seamlessly from chapter to chapter and from disease to disease, highlighting how injury to one part affects other parts, and the whole body. This makes for easy reading. I would recommend this book to my patients and interested colleagues.
Emmanuel Quaye, MD

If you want to learn more about how to better care for yourself, pick up this book.
Carol Lee Hilewick, PhD

In this excellent book, Dr. Luis Arrondo draws on his clinical experiences and on extensive research in the scientific literature to reveal important connections for any person wanting to achieve better health.
Jorge Rivera-Diaz, MD

Dr. Arrondo integrates his clinical expertise and thorough research to provide deep insight into the interconnections of bodily functions, mind and spirit as they play critical roles in maintaining and enhancing health. Each chapter offers practical suggestions for maximizing health through self care and, when necessary, working effectively with health-care providers. For anyone wishing to maintain optimal health, this is an extremely valuable resource. I am grateful for the wisdom he shares.
Carol Ames, MS

I am thrilled to have an easy-to-understand guide that shows us at deeper levels how the human body works together to heal. I would recommend this book in and out of my classroom.
Linda Duerson, Health Education Instructor

Whether you want to address a health concern or maintain optimal health, you'll find solutions in *Wolves, Gardens, and Chocolate.*
Peg Stirn, RN, BCB

Wolves, Gardens, and Chocolate

WOLVES, GARDENS, AND CHOCOLATE

THE LITTLE-KNOWN CONNECTIONS TO VIBRANT HEALTH, IDEAL WEIGHT, AND BOUNDLESS ENERGY

INCLUDES OVER 900 SCIENTIFIC RESEARCH CITATIONS

Luis Arrondo, DC

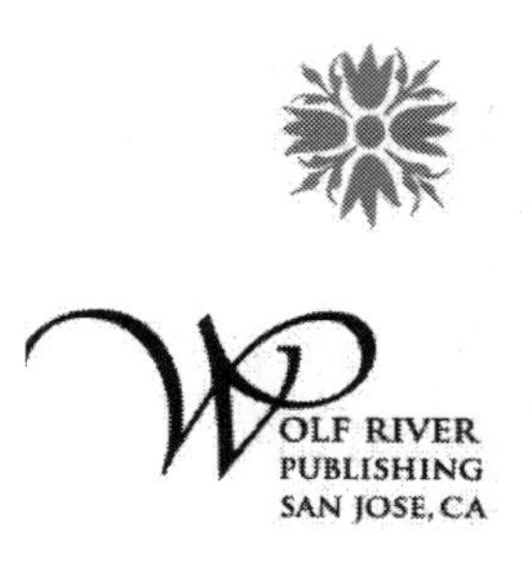

Wolves, Gardens, and Chocolate: The Little-Known Connections to Vibrant Health, Ideal Weight, and Boundless Energy

Wolf River Publishing
1101 S. Winchester Blvd. Suite J-210
San Jose, California, 95128.

Quantity sales: Special discounts are available on quantity purchases by corporations, associations, and others. For details, contact the publisher's address above.

This book, with narrative additions, is also available in Spanish, titled *Tu cuerpo es un jardín: Cómo tu cuerpo **realmente** funciona.*

Design by Chris Molé
Editing by Elissa Rabellino
Author photograph by David Turner Photography
First printing 2016

Printed in the United States of America.

Arrondo, Luis.

Wolves, Gardens, and Chocolate: The Little-Known Connections to Vibrant Health, Ideal Weight, and Boundless Energy / Luis Arrondo, DC.

p. cm.

"Includes over 900 Scientific Research Citations"
ISBN 978-0-9966065-0-9 print book
ISBN 978-0-9966065-1-6 eBook
Includes bibliographical references and index.

1. Integrative medicine. 2. Holistic medicine. 3. Alternative medicine. 4. Health. 5. Mind and body. 6. Nutrition. I. Title.

RA776.5 .A77 2015

613 --dc23 2015915358

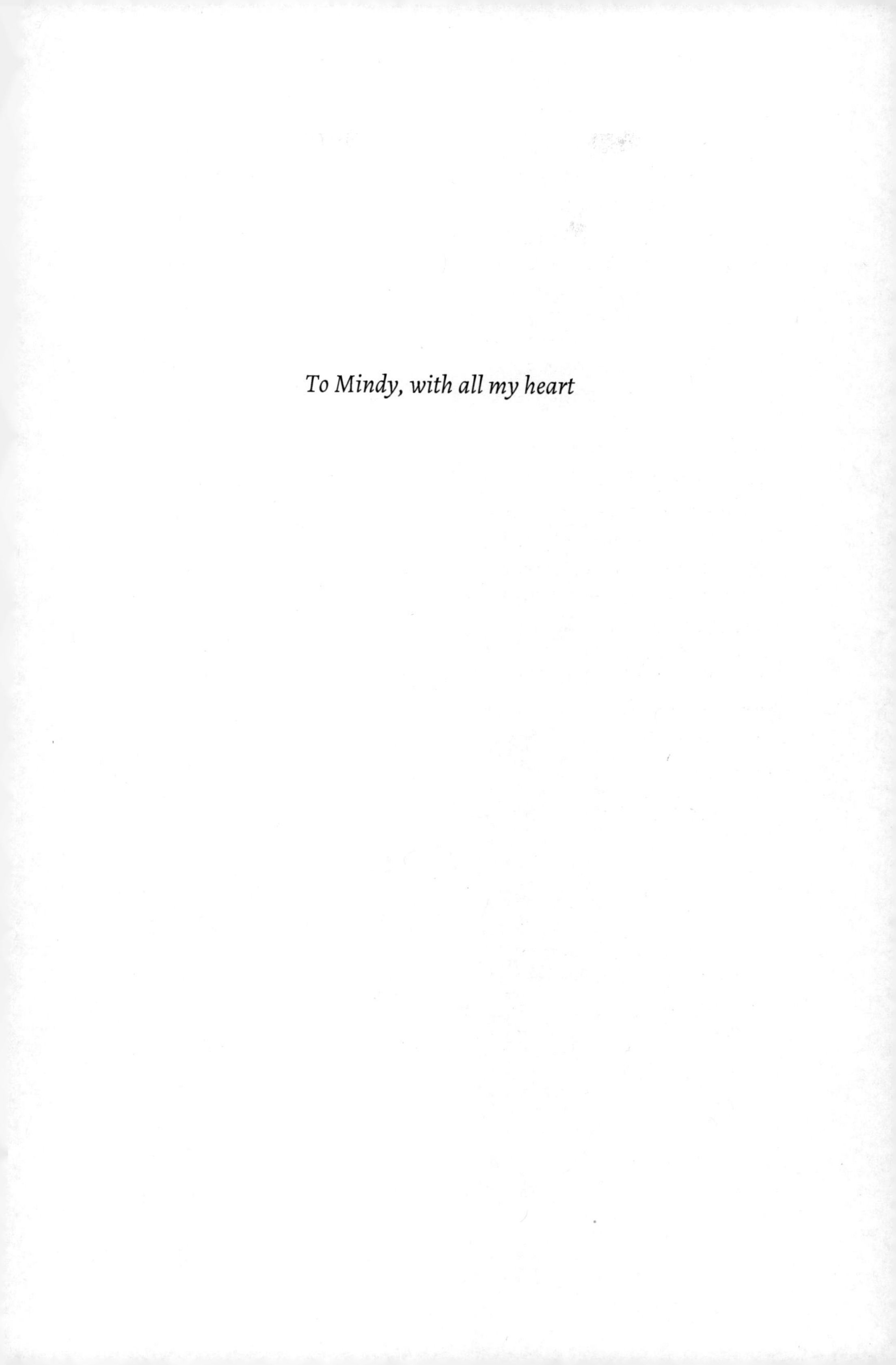

To Mindy, with all my heart

Contents

DISCLAIMER AND NOTICES

Limit of liability/disclaimer of Warranty:

The contents of this book are presented as an informational source for appropriate consideration by readers and their treating physicians. It is not to be used for diagnostic or treatment purposes. It does not create a patient-physician relationship. It should not be used as a substitute for any professional diagnosis or treatment, whether physical, mental, or of any other type. The contents of this book are presented with the intention of helping to bring awareness of nutritionally significant information as well as other types of information, including suggestions and protocols that readers can discuss with their treating physicians.

Information about the use of nutritional supplements and other natural approaches is not offered to replace established medical approaches. Rather, this book serves to present topics of discussion between patients and their doctors. The contents of this book, including the discussion of nutritional and other health approaches, are not a substitute for the advice of a treating health professional and should not be construed as an attempt to offer or render a medical opinion or otherwise engage in the practice of medicine. It is not meant, nor should it be used, to diagnose, treat, cure, or prevent disease. The author cannot be held responsible for any information, omissions, or errors, inadvertent or otherwise, contained herein. The user of this information has the sole responsibility of determining if any of the information provided in this book is appropriate. It is recommended in all cases that the user consult a licensed doctor with the appropriate scope of practice to make this determination. No medical, legal, or professional services are offered.

Please consult your health care provider before making any health care decisions or for guidance about a specific condition. The author and publisher of this book expressly disclaim responsibility and shall have no liability for any loss, injury, or damage, whether consequential, incidental, or special, or of any other type, as a result of your reliance on the information contained in this book or its use. This book gives information on, but does not endorse specifically, any test, treatment, or procedure mentioned on the site. The information contained herein is provided without any representations or warranties, express or implied.

This book was written and researched solely by Luis Arrondo, D.C.

When one tugs at a single thing in nature,
one finds it attached to the rest of the world.

—John Muir, naturalist, 1838–1914

The physician is the servant of nature, not her master.
Therefore, it behooves the physician to follow the will of nature.

—Paracelsus, physician, 1493–1541

Introduction

I AM INSPIRED and humbled by my patients every day.

Most of them work long hours. Some have more than one job to make ends meet. Their bodies are failing them in a number of ways—some for many years. Many are frustrated, anxious, confused, wondering if they will ever feel well again. They've lost the sweet fruit of good health that they had when they were younger, and they yearn for it again.

For more than 20 years as a doctor of chiropractic, I have helped sick people recover from chronic illnesses, many in a relatively short period of time.

As the years unfolded, I discovered the profound effect of sharing with my patients my observations as well as the research that brought to light the connections between seemingly unrelated bodily functions and my patients' abilities to heal. These were hidden connections that affected, either to their benefit or their detriment, their capacity to recuperate, to feel better, and to have more energy. Here was a vital network of exciting healing opportunities that they became aware of and started to apply.

I helped my patients to understand the connections between their conditions and how the rest of their body worked, and about connections that could either help or hurt their chances of getting better. As a result, they began to experience how paying attention to the well-being of seemingly unrelated body systems helped them to become healthier and have less pain.

Wolves, Gardens, and Chocolate will help you to take easy, logical steps toward better health from a perspective that you may have never considered. As you will see from examples, getting the big picture and looking at your body from an expanded, integrated sense of how it really works is often the most important aspect of attaining good health.

Explore how your condition can serve as a valuable learning experience about your deepest self. Revisit ancient cultures that worked with the meaning of dreams, and learn how dreams can help to heal you. Understand how your life's purpose and expression can be intimately connected to your health, or lack of it, and what you can do to help yourself. Begin to experience your body and your health from a new, expanded perspective.

If you are in ill health, this book can help you learn how to have more energy, achieve better health, and finally get to your desired weight, without going hungry. After all, if you want different results, you need to start to think and to act differently! The joyful surprise that my patients express when their health issues start to resolve after years of frustration and pain can be your experience as well.

We need to move beyond the traditional clinical perspective, one that is usually microscopic in application, and to open more widely the doors of curiosity and acceptance, embracing a more expansive, telescopic view of health. A greater openness to explore the diversity of healing paradigms, some of them much older than Western science, others new and emerging, can help more clinicians to benefit from the breadth and clinical wisdom of other cultures. This will enable more patients to achieve better health, in all its aspects.

As you will see, getting the big picture and looking at your body from an expanded sense of how it really works is often the most important aspect of attaining good health. Doing so will help you to work in greater awareness of how your body can finally heal.

In *Wolves, Gardens, and Chocolate,* I will explain this network of connections. For those who have a deeper interest in the research, there are more than 900 scientific citations, grouped by chapter, at the end of the text. At the end of each chapter is a section called "What You Can Do Now," which contains quick, practical suggestions and information related to the topics covered in the chapter.

Most books on health are divided into sections. I refrained from doing so, since one of the messages of this book is that to attain better health at all levels we need to stop treating and dividing our body into parts, or sections, and to explore more deeply the connections of the seemingly unrelated as a tool to healing.

The way in which I wrote this book reflects this, and so does the title. Nothing is neatly all in one place, because that is not how our bodies function, nor how they heal. The book's underlying rhythm and introduction of topics are designed to aid you to a deeper recognition about your health.

One of these patterns is central to the theme of the book, and runs from the first chapter to the last: The book begins with a discussion of the weaknesses in our health care, then highlights our biological connections while illustrating throughout the book how the emotional, mental, and spiritual aspects of our life are so closely intertwined with how health expresses itself.

For those, however, who would like to focus on a topic or a condition, the detailed index in the back and the short and easy-to-access chapters with descriptive subheadings in the Contents will serve that purpose.

It is my hope to provide you with tools to help you gain a greater clarity about your symptoms, yourself, and perhaps your purpose in life.

A spirit of open inquiry, of stretching your thoughts, and of expanding how you see things is perhaps the most enduring sign of a thriving garden of good health.

It's time for a change.

Change starts with you.

[1]

A Patient's Frustration

"DOC, HERE'S MY story: I'm 39 years old, but I feel like I'm 50! I've gained 20 pounds in the last 10 years. My neck and back ache, I don't have much energy, I don't sleep well, and I feel bloated after eating. I also get headaches in the afternoon and during my menstrual periods."

I quietly listened to the patient. It was her first visit to my clinic, and she was eager to vent some of her frustrations. "On top of that, my sex life with my husband isn't good, and I get tired at work. One of my children has been gaining weight and isn't doing well in school. I'm losing hope."

She fidgeted uncomfortably as she counted off the prescriptions and natural supplements she had taken throughout the years. According to her, nothing had made a significant difference. It was evident to me that she had been searching for a long time to find a way to turn a corner on her chronic health issues.

After going over the issues that she had listed on her intake form, I paused and asked, "It seems to me that your garden isn't doing well, is it?"

She gave me a puzzled look. "My garden? I'm not talking about my backyard, Doctor. I'm talking about my health. Why a garden?"

"Your health and your body are like a garden," I responded. "Start thinking of treating your health and your body the way that you would a garden. It will help you to understand more deeply how your body works and heals."

I observed her carefully. Her appearance was that of a tired, overweight middle-aged woman facing more problems than foreseeable solutions. The frustration on her face was typical of a pattern that I frequently see at the clinic—men and women who have experienced years of varying degrees of health dysfunction, with no end in sight.

I suggested that if she started to view herself and her health differently, it would be easier for her to make the changes she was looking for. I was confident that a different approach could bring different results for her.

Sometimes offering a simple metaphor can help a patient to experience a new viewpoint and act in ways that help improve many underlying health issues.

Step back for a moment, and look at how your body works from a different perspective. Consider looking at your body as a garden, as though you were a master gardener in charge of maintaining a healthy assortment of plants, flowers, fruits, and vegetables. We could learn a lot about our own health by observing the way a master gardener cultivates his garden.

When master gardeners attend to their gardens, perhaps looking at bright red rows of strawberries, or tomatoes hanging lazily from bright green vines, they don't immediately apply a chemical, or even a natural compound, if they observe that parts of the garden have turned yellow or some plants have wilted.

They are aware that there are a lot of reasons why a plant, or perhaps the entire garden, might not be healthy. What might help one plant could be bad for another with a similar condition; sometimes a yellow leaf can be a result of not enough water—or too much.

Our health problems are like those yellow leaves; the root causes can be quite different from person to person, even if they have similar symptoms. A master gardener looks for connections underlying the problems and then seeks to find the root causes.

We should be doing the same with our health.

A garden is composed of solid soil, yet above it, in the lightness of the air, the rain, wind, and sun are essential to it. In parallel fashion, the root causes of many of our health problems can lie beyond the cells and tissues of our bodies. Exploring the connections between health, healing, and illnesses, and our worlds of perceptions, emotions, actions, dreams, memories, and thoughts can be profoundly revealing, as well as necessary to bring more profound healing.

Throughout this book, beginning with an emphasis on the physical processes in our bodies, we will explore experiences and research about the emotional, mental, and spiritual aspects of ourselves that can lead not only to better health, but also to the opportunity to live with greater fulfillment.

After all, a master gardener also looks up.

After I explained this to my patient, she looked at me intently, pausing for a long, uncertain moment, as if she was making up her mind. Then she said that she agreed, saying that she wanted to move out of her rut of taking prescriptions for her symptoms or following the latest wonder drug or health product on TV, on the Internet, or in magazines. The frustration in her voice, however, was evident.

And I wasn't surprised.

What You Can Do Now

- Look at your health as more than a set of parts that need be chemically balanced. Think of your body not as a car, with interchangeable pieces, but as a connected, integrated ecosystem, like a garden. As you go through this book, consider and reflect on all of the dynamics, at all levels, that could be involved with your persistent health issues.

[2]

Health Care: Beware the Hidden Risks

IN FACT, MANY people share her frustration and are going through a similar situation. The United States is home to roughly 315 million people, including infants and young children. In one year, more than four billion prescriptions—not over-the-counter remedies or natural supplements, but actual prescriptions—are filled, and that number continues to increase annually.[1] That's an average of 13 prescriptions a year for every American.

The population of the United States represents approximately 5 percent of the world's population, and yet we account for 75 percent of the world's prescriptions.[2] So it takes, on average, the annual prescriptions of 57 people worldwide to reach the annual prescription average for each American.

Are we really that sick?

Every prescription drug is known to have approximately 70 possible side effects, on average. Multiply that by 13 prescriptions a year, and you have the possibility of a great number of side effects, many overlapping, that the average patient and his or her prescribing doctor need to be aware of.[3]

How many people end up in the hospital yearly due to the use of prescribed drugs?

More than two million visits are made to emergency rooms each year in the U.S. due to the use of prescription medication—even taken as prescribed. Over 100,000 deaths occur in this country yearly as a result of adverse drug reactions.[4,5]

Almost half of all Americans are on at least one prescription drug. And the number of Americans taking five or more prescription drugs has doubled in the past 10 years.[6]

Let's explore some of the reasons for those stunning statistics and what they could mean to you if you are, or will be, taking prescription medications.

First I want to go over how a prescription drug works and how its function may vary from person to person. The same drug dosage may also affect you differently at various times in your life. Why? Because drugs typically work by activating receptors in your cells. That is known as the *drug action.* How your body responds to that is known as the *drug effect,* and that can vary.

All drugs basically go through four steps, or processes, called *pharmacokinetics.* Drugs are first absorbed, then distributed within your body, metabolized, and finally excreted.

However, not every one of the steps works the same for each person, or for the same person at all times. Not everyone's digestive system can absorb nutrients or medications as well as others. When drugs are distributed within your body and you have edema, you may need a bigger dose at times—or less if you are dehydrated. If you are very obese, some drugs don't distribute well to fatty tissues.

Most drugs are metabolized in the liver. People whose liver is not working well may need a dosage that is different from others. Some people metabolize drugs in their liver very quickly, so patients are classified according to how quickly they metabolize drugs. This rate affects what a patient's dosage should be, and drug toxicity can result if the dosage is incorrect for that patient.

The body handles excretion of drugs in different ways. Your kidneys do most of the work. Those who have kidney challenges may not be able to get rid of the residues of the drugs as well as others, which also leads to drug toxicity.

Other factors come into play when considering how a person will react to a drug. Age is one of them. Older people typically have less muscle mass, and their kidneys usually do not work as well as when they were middle-aged or younger. They would usually need lower dosages or risk drug-toxicity issues. Diet and digestive issues can lead to malnutrition, which can affect the number of proteins in the blood available to bind with the medicine, influencing how the medicine is used by the body.

Polymorphism, a type of genetic variation common in the population, is studied in the expanding field of pharmacogenetics. It can also affect how you will respond to a drug, especially when variations for proteins named *cytochrome isoenzymes* are found. Approximately one-third of all medications are metabolized by the cytochrome P450 system.

As you can see, there are a lot of variables with any medication you take. Keep in mind that many side effects are still not known. As research continues, we have become aware, for example, of more side effects involved with statin drugs.

People who have no blood sugar issues and are in good health are likely to become up to two and a half times more susceptible to type 2 diabetes when statins, used for cholesterol and more recently for cardiovascular issues, are prescribed.[7] For those who are already diabetic, new research is showing that statin use is associated with very high risks of diabetic complications.[8]

Prescription drugs in many cases play an important role, saving and prolonging lives. However, since they can also be dangerous, I suggest that my patients use them as little as clinically reasonable. With the increasing number of drugs available, it's important to consult with your prescribing physician (in addition to researching on your own) as to a medication's merits and side effects.

I explained to my patient that although the aging population accounted for part of the reason why prescription rates have increased so much in the past 10 years, the number of prescriptions for the younger generation has also risen.

Let's explore some of the reasons behind this growth, and its dangers to your health.

An Adversarial Approach to Illness

Our common approach to illness is usually adversarial. With the introduction of wonderful chemical tools, our everyday language includes phrases such as "I'm fighting this," or "I'm killing that," or "the war against"—even if the diseases were caused by our lifestyle decisions.

It's an approach, weaknesses and strengths aside, that has an important place in the clinical toolbox, saving countless lives, and improving many others.

There are a number of reasons for an adversarial approach, many based on tradition and culture. One of the challenges has to do with the usual clinical approach to illness. One of the primary goals for physicians is to establish a diagnosis—in other words, give a name or pathology to the condition or illness. The next step physicians usually take is to find a drug or drugs that best treat that illness.

The process typically involves looking for the offending agent—say, a strain of bacteria—and introducing powerful chemicals to kill it. This approach has been much more effective since antibiotics became widely available to the general public after the end of World War II.

Chronic or long-term health conditions, however, are often the result of complex processes due to challenges in how the body regulates itself. It is not always an infectious issue. Additionally, areas that aren't symptomatic might be affecting other parts or functions that do show symptoms.

Most of the time, before a chronic illness is initially diagnosed, our body hasn't functioned well for a long time. The changes might have been subtle, but our body's ability to heal itself was compromised.

Think of it like a gas tank with a slow leak: over time, the gas level drops unnoticed until the "empty" light blinks on, or worse, you find yourself stranded out on the highway without gas. A lot of people feel that they are already running on fumes!

Health Care's Paradigm

Our health care system is effective at, and emphasizes, crisis management. A health care system that works within this paradigm can be compared to waiting until the "empty" light on your car's dashboard begins to glow before taking a closer look at what's going on.

Our health care system, however, is slow to pick up signs that there is a problem with the proverbial gas tank before you are left stranded somewhere.

By the time you are given a diagnosis, treatment is usually handled through a chemical approach: prescriptions based on presenting symptoms and signs.

Our bodies, however, are so complex and interconnected that proper functioning of one part is dependent on how everything else is working. That means there are patients who exhibit a similar set of symptoms that have different causes.

Most people don't give much thought to the clinical parameters that have been used when treating them or their loved ones. Symptom-focused clinical approaches have benefits, but they also have limitations that we need to consider.

Some segments of modern medicine are beginning to recognize this deeper network of causes and effects in the body, exploring the multisystem connections that have caused chronic illness. Examples are the emerging fields of network biology and network pharmacology, which are arising from the realization that sticking to a one-disease, one-drug approach is a clinical paradigm that is limited and needs to be changed.[9,10]

The health care system is set up so that you go see a doctor when you don't feel well. Doctors are trained to look for pathology, or diseases, and then recommend a course of action, usually pharmacological in nature, which can be lifesaving.

This leads to health care that is largely chemically based, through prescriptions, which are given in 80 percent of all office visits. This approach obviously offers a number of benefits, including saving many lives. However, the ability to receive the best health care possible is limited when the usual approach is illness-based and chemically driven.

What we are receiving is actually sickness care. You typically go to a hospital because you are sick or because you are suspected of having a serious illness. We wait until we are sick before going to a place to better our health: we have illness-based hospitals.

A Different Viewpoint

To change this approach, we must first change our point of view. Why not consider having wellness-based hospitals and healing centers? Places where healthy people can go to improve whatever level of health they are at so they don't end up in doctors' waiting rooms.

We have gyms and spas, so why don't we have this wellness approach in our hospitals?

Our society views health as the absence of disease, but in reality, our bodies do not function in a simple black-and-white manner. Our health conditions are fluid and dynamic, and flow along the lines of a spectrum. The closer you are toward the healthy end of the spectrum, the less likely you are to have diseases and the more likely you are to experience and enjoy the fullness of life.

I learned early on in my practice that placing an emphasis on educating my patients was an integral part of the treatment process. With the right knowledge, an inquisitive, informed patient can sidestep areas of weakness in our health care delivery system and maximize its strengths.

This book will give you insights in how to do that, at every level of your life.

We should keep in mind that these facts highlight systemic rather than individual deficiencies. Every branch of the proverbial tree of healing includes men and women earnestly striving to provide the best clinical care they can. It's the system that is slow to adapt and change. In fact, that's the way it has always been with large, institutionalized clinical approaches.

UNNECESSARY ANTIBIOTICS

Let's take a look at the type of prescription most patients need to be more informed about: antibiotics. Research shows how strongly antibiotic prescriptions are being overused, with negative consequences for current and future generations.

Approximately 260 million prescriptions are written every year for antibiotics in the U.S.; that's almost one prescription annually for every adult. According to an article in the *New England Journal of Medicine,* as many as 50 percent of those prescriptions are unnecessary.[11]

It's a case-by-case call, and there are always exceptions, but generally speaking, many of the antibiotics that are prescribed for bronchitis, acute ear infections, and typical sore throat cases are unnecessary.

A study published in the *Journal of General Internal Medicine,* noted below, showed that the correct use of antibiotics in acute bronchitis should be "close to zero." However:

- The national rate of antibiotic prescriptions is approximately 73 percent.[12]
- For sore throats, antibiotic prescriptions are usually needed 10 percent of the time, when strep is an issue.
- The national average prescription rate for sore throats is, however, 60 percent.[13]

You might ask, what's the big deal—isn't it better to be safe than sorry? Let's take a close look at this issue. Overuse of antibiotics might be adding to the dramatic increases in obesity, allergies, diabetes, and inflammatory bowel disease.[14,15]

The more people use antibiotics, the greater the likelihood that they will develop type 2 diabetes. If five or more prescriptions were filled in a 12-year period, the risk of developing diabetes was 53 percent higher than those that did not use any.[16]

This excessive use of antibiotics has contributed to what is called *the post-antibiotic era*. Each year, more than two million people in the United States are infected with bacteria that are resistant to antibiotics.[17] In fact, the Centers for Disease Control is running an active campaign to help physicians correctly prescribe antibiotics.[18]

Antibiotics are becoming less effective due in large part to their indiscriminate use. Almost half of infections related to common surgeries are due to pathogens that are resistant to the usual antibiotics.[19,20]

Urinary tract infections, or UTIs, are a common problem for many women, especially when they involve recurrent infections. One reason this is occurring more frequently is that they have antibiotic-resistant organisms that have not been eliminated through antibiotic prescriptions. Excessive use of antibiotics has also been an issue here, leading to antibiotic-resistant strains.

Bacteria that cause UTIs are known as *uropathogens*. Most UTIs are caused by bacteria. In one study, over half of 166 uropathogens were shown to have a high degree of resistance to multiple antibiotics.[21] A simple herbal extract, however, was proven to be effective in a laboratory setting against most of these multi-drug-resistant pathogens.[22] I will discuss more about this in chapter 3.

There are other concerns. Many UTIs are misdiagnosed. Some sexually transmitted diseases, known as STDs, can show the same type of urine lab test results as UTIs, as well as similar symptoms, including urgent, painful, and frequent urination.[23] There are 65 million Americans living with an STD. Of those, over one million women each year contract chlamydia, the most commonly reported STD in the country. It is most often seen in young women. If you have recurring UTIs, considering asking your doctor to consider doing STD testing when you have a urinalysis. Many males have it without knowing it or experiencing symptoms, and can continue to infect their partners.

We discussed the connection between antibiotics and diabetes; let's turn our attention to a topic that few would typically consider: is there a connection between obesity and antibiotics? Think about this: could the increased use of antibiotics have contributed to the fact that the average American weighs 24 pounds more than he or she did three decades ago?[24]

There is concern that several rounds of antibiotics may increase the weight and bone growth of children, with effects lasting throughout adulthood. One study was based on antibiotics usually prescribed for children that were administered to mice. The study also revealed that the balance and number of beneficial bacteria in the gut was also affected.[25] Other studies have come up with similar results, suggesting that gut microbial changes may alter how food is absorbed.

The average child in America undergoes 10 rounds of antibiotics by the age of 10.

Antibiotics have been used to help livestock gain significant amounts of weight. Research has also shown that giving antibiotics to children or adults increases their weight, even when they always eat the same amount of calories. The issue might be particularly dramatic for women. When researchers studied female rats that were given antibiotics, there was a much greater increase in the percentage of fat gained, compared with the male rats. But the weight of both genders in that study increased when compared with the rats that ate the same amount of food without being given antibiotics.[26]

Young mice that were given antibiotics had a greater chance of becoming obese as adults. It seems that antibiotics change the population of the bacteria in the intestines so that the metabolic rate is slowed.[27]

Most of the antibiotics produced in the United States, almost 30 million pounds per year, are used for livestock. This contributes to an increase in antibiotic-resistant organisms. It is hard to isolate control groups of humans for long-term research who are certain to have never ingested antibiotics through the food chain. Additional research will be helpful but perhaps never definitive.

My point is that patients will be served best by keeping their eyes open, inquiring, and being willing to look at the usual differently.

We are working with a health care system that has wonderful physicians, nurses, and practitioners of every type. However, the system shows strengths and weaknesses, patterns of strong concern that can affect your health and that of your family. As a result, you have to become more aware of these patterns. In the end, you are responsible for your health.

I mentioned earlier that 80 percent of all doctor visits in the United States result in prescribed drug therapy.[28] It's evidence of a largely monolithic approach that does not fully serve our health needs.

Doctors often feel pressure from patients to overprescribe. In an effort to change that, a study was conducted in which physicians promised in writing not to prescribe antibiotics that were more harmful than helpful to their patients. That promise was posted on the walls of clinics so that patients could see it. The efforts resulted in modestly decreased unnecessary prescription rates.[29]

Another factor in overprescribing is geographical. Researchers have found that doctors in some southern states prescribe twice as many antibiotics as doctors along the West Coast, per 1,000 patients of all ages. There are no disease-specific variations in these regions to account for the different rates.

The variation extends to other drugs as well and is part of a bigger pattern. Some states in the South prescribe almost three times as many opioid painkillers per 100 patients as states in the West.[30] Sales of opioid pain relievers have increased threefold in less than 12 years, enough to medicate every adult in America with a typical dosage every four hours, continuously, for a month.[31,32]

What's more, painkillers are prescribed twice as often per person in the United States as in Canada.[33]

If you go to Paris for your summer vacation or honeymoon and get sick, keep in mind that antibiotics are prescribed over three times as often there per 1,000 patients than if you spent those hot August days exploring the fjords of Norway.[34]

Recently, the top-selling drug in America, with over $7 billion in sales, was an antipsychotic drug, Abilify.

Women patients in America are at particular risk for receiving too many prescriptions. Over 25 percent of them have a prescription for a mental health drug.[35] The rate for men is around 15 percent.

Next time you stand at the checkout line in the supermarket or are in line at the movies, look around and count. One out of every four women in that line, statistically speaking, is on a prescription for a mental health drug.[36] Areas of the country where the incidence of diabetes is higher, such as the "diabetes belt" in certain southern states, have increased rates of mental health prescriptions due to higher levels of anxiety and depression among diabetics.

Surgical Interventions: Location Matters

The discrepancies in clinical approaches don't stop with drugs. Surgery rates for the same procedure can be up to four times more frequent in one region of the United States than in another, not because there are more conditions or diseases in that area that need that type of surgery, but because of geographical differences in approaches. According to the authors of one national study, the decision to operate might depend strongly on where you live, not just on the doctor, or the illness or injury.[37]

For example, patients in surgical teaching hospitals in Salt Lake City are twice as likely to get knee-replacement surgery as patients in teaching hospitals in Manhattan. Back surgery in Nashville in surgical teaching hospitals occurs almost three times more often than in teaching hospitals in Philadelphia, and lower-extremity bypass surgery rates in teaching hospitals in Baltimore are over twice the U.S. average for teaching hospitals. On a global scale, spinal surgery rates in the United States are five times higher than in Britain and twice as high as in Canada and Europe.[38,39]

Sometimes whether surgery is performed or not extends beyond geography. It can vary depending on what type of practitioner a patient sees first. In a study involving 1,885 injured workers in the state of Washington with low back pain over a three-year period, those who saw a chiropractor first ended up with lumbar surgery 1.5 percent of the time. Those who saw a surgeon first had low-back surgery 42.7 percent of the time. The researchers stated that there was very strong association between surgery rates and the type of first provider seen, even after adjusting for other important variables.[40]

At other times surgery is performed with the expectation that it will help the patient, although the science for predicting successful outcomes may be lacking. Chronic low back pain is one of the biggest causes of disability throughout the world. There is no medically known anatomical cause. For many, spinal fusion surgery is a suggested option, and for many, it has been of help. There is no evidence, however, of any prognostic test for chronic low back pain that points to spinal fusion as reliable or effective treatment.[41]

How medicine is practiced is neither as scientific nor as consistent as you might think.

There are a lot of gray areas in every specialty. After all, the word *medicine* comes from the Latin for "the art of healing." In Cecil's *Textbook of Medicine, medicine* is defined as a profession that incorporates science and scientific methods with the art of being a physician.[42]

Medicine is an art that integrates the application of a changing and sometimes contradictory scientific process along with the personal experiences and insights of each physician. Less than half of the practice of medicine is supported by research.[43,44]

The inconsistencies go beyond clinical treatments and into the foundation of clinical research that is used to support health protocols.

It takes approximately 17 years for clinical research to find its way into daily clinical practice.[45,46,47,48,49]

Approximately one-third of highly cited research found in mainstream medical journals is later either contradicted or shown to have findings that were not accurate.[50,51,52] The system in place that ensures that biomedical research is reproducible is failing, according the U.S. National Institutes of Health.[53]

This is a problem that extends to all disciplines of health, including psychology, where more than half of the findings of research papers published did not hold up under further review by other researchers.[54]

Doctors are doing the best they can, but it's the system itself that needs changing. The authors involved in some research noted above also suggested that patients should speak more openly with their doctors.

I like to share with my patients that they will be served best by keeping their eyes open, inquiring, and being willing to look at conventional wisdom differently. Prescription drugs, obviously, should be taken when necessary. However, drugs, and surgery if needed, should be the last resort, not necessarily the first line of treatment.

Now let's explore some of the challenges found in the present health care system with examining patients, a critical part of leading to diagnosis and treatment.

Doctors have a wonderful array of modern analytical and technical tools with which to diagnose and treat their patients. However, it has been suggested that doctors also need to return to a more physical approach, using their knowledge and abilities to examine the patient personally, as doctors did in the past.[55,56,57] Studies published in the *New England Journal of Medicine* and in the *American Journal of Medicine,* as well as in other journals, show that ever since the rise of modern medical technology in the 1980s, basic, hands-on physical examination skills have eroded.[58,59,60,61,62,63]

There's more compelling research on why doctors should stop relying so strongly on medical technology. According to the National Academy of Medicine, one-third of health care expenditures don't improve the health of patients.[64,65,66] Research shows that up to 40 percent of all CT scans ordered are not necessary.[67,68,69] CT scans involve high doses of ionizing radiation. The Food and Drug Administration has warned that large numbers of people are receiving CT scans that are of uncertain benefit due to radiation-associated cancer risks.[70]

Other challenges within our health system that can have an effect on how you will be treated have to do with external forces, which are increasing each year.

Doctors are under a lot of pressure these days from various sectors: financial, administrative, insurance companies, and even patients. Over one-third of physicians are willing to order tests that they know are unnecessary if the patient insists. These pressures put a stress on the capacity to deliver optimal health care, despite the earnest efforts of caring and qualified physicians and nurses. The opposite is true as well, to the detriment of the patient. Tests or treatment that insurance companies won't pay for are often not performed.

There have been changes in recent years in the financial structure of many medical practices that also pose a risk to the health of patients, and which can alter which procedures they undergo. Many hospitals and corporations are hiring doctors at an increased rate. More and more, economic relationships are being established between doctors, labs, ambulatory surgical centers, imaging centers, and hospitals.

But would that make a difference in your care, you might ask? According to a report published by the Government Accountability Office, it can make a big difference. This physician self-referral report revealed that physicians or their families who have a financial interest in these types of arrangements benefit financially by ordering more tests and procedures.[71]

When doctors enter into a financial relationship with them, the percentage of patients that they refer for imaging and procedures jumps up dramatically. Advanced imaging studies, such as MRI (*magnetic resonance imaging*) and CT scans, jumped by 66 percent within two years. Differences in these numbers were not explained by age, gender, health status, or geography. Requests for biopsies after doctors entered into financial arrangements with pathology services companies increased between 18 and 56 percent compared with the order rate of doctors that did not have any financial ties.[72,73]

Recommendation for radiation therapy for prostate cancer patients increased by over 50 percent when the doctor started to benefit financially. At the same time, more conservative measures, such as active surveillance, decreased 8 percent. So did the rates of recommendation for other, less invasive treatments.

In none of the instances above could the differences be accounted for by age, beneficiary health, or geographic location, according to the government report.

Surgery rates among doctors who have financial ties with ambulatory surgery centers increased more rapidly than among doctors who did not.[74]

Financial ties are one reason why medical radiation exposure has increased by a factor of seven in the past 35 years. Up to 2 percent of all cancers may be due to radiation exposure.[75]

Here is one thing to consider doing about it. Next time a test, procedure, or surgery is suggested, ask the doctor if he or any family member has any financial relationship with the provider of services. You now know that there is a greater chance that unnecessary testing or procedures may take place when the doctor in some way reaps financial benefits from recommending them. I will mention a resource to get consensus opinions from other groups of doctors later in this chapter.

The nature of hospital care is, by itself, another risk to consider. One-third of hospitalized patients are harmed during their stay, and as many as 98,000 die in hospitals each year due to preventable medical errors.[76,77,78]

A number of doctors have been finding themselves at odds with insurance companies and hospital administrators because of the introduction of monitoring procedures and financial pressures that help to contain costs but might not serve the best interests of the patient.

Increasingly, many doctors are monitored to measure what testing and treatment they use for their patients, and the cost. With the introduction of sophisticated analyses, administrators can measure how many tests each doctor is ordering and track the test results for the doctor's patient base. Insurers give a bonus to these doctors if they meet establish clinical goals for the patients.

Not all patients benefit equally from the same numbers-driven approach. For some, it could be to their detriment. The history of individual reactions to certain types of medications might indicate that less aggressive pharmaceutical approaches would serve a patient best. Yet doctors who deviate from this numbers-based approach could receive lower pay or stop being preferentially listed on insurers' websites.[79]

Financial pressure is now becoming a factor in what medications a doctor will prescribe. For some doctors, choosing a certain treatment plan chosen by the insurance company will result in a paid monthly bonus.[80]

On the one hand, I appreciate insurers' efforts at cost containment and uniformity. The challenge, however, is that a group-driven approach is being used, while every person is different. These facts, and more to follow, point to patients' needing to play a more active role in advocating for their health.

C-Sections: Pressures and Risks

Taking into account what we've covered so far, it's ironic to point out that there are times when uniformity in the health care system is, indeed, not always a good sign. When man first landed on the moon in 1969, approximately 4 in 100 women gave birth via cesarean section. That number now has risen to almost 1 in 3 women.[81,82,83]

C-section has become the most common surgical procedure in U.S. hospitals, although less than 1 percent of women request a cesarean section without a medical reason.[84] Research indicates, however, that giving birth by cesarean delivery solely due to medical reasons is between 5 and 10 percent.[85,86,87]

Sometimes cesarean delivery not only is the best choice but also can be lifesaving. However, that's a decision that a patient needs to carefully consider with her obstetrician before going through with the procedure. Keep in mind that there are financial pressures regarding birth by C-section, as well as matters of convenience, medical malpractice issues, and time.

Almost one-third of obstetricians who participated in a survey admitted that they were performing more C-sections due to fear of a lawsuit. And up to one-quarter of all women have reported experiencing pressure to have a C-section rather than natural delivery.[88]

Since the majority of C-sections are not predicated by medical need, it's wise for any expectant mother to be aware that along with any benefits that delivery by C-section might provide, there can also be disadvantages to the health of the mother and the child.

Infections acquired by the mother are more common with C-sections, along with complications that can affect the mother, such as placenta implantation problems and an increased need for a hysterectomy.

The way a baby is born can also have a long-term effect on the health of the child.

When a natural delivery takes place, movement through the vaginal canal helps populate the baby's gastrointestinal tract with beneficial bacterial flora. In a C-section, the baby instead has flora in his gastrointestinal tract seeded by the bacteria found on the skin of the mother, which is not the same beneficial type. The development of the correct types and amounts of beneficial bacteria in the intestines, which constitutes an important part of the immune system, is altered.[89]

The importance of healthy gut flora in a young child is hard to overemphasize. Breastfeeding is the best way to introduce these beneficial bacteria. Breastfed children are less likely to suffer from obesity and diabetes later in life.[90]

Bacteria from the mother affect the child in more profound ways than most people realize. The common assumption is that a child's traits come from the DNA of the parents. However, it has recently been discovered that a mother's bacteria also influence the traits of her offspring in ways that were previously thought to happen only through DNA.[91]

A growing number of children are experiencing issues with allergies and inflammatory disorders. Delivery by C-section versus vaginal delivery has been found to modify the workings of the immune system and the physiology of the gut. Children born by C-section can experience greater amounts of chronic disorders, including inflammatory bowel disease. Research also points to a relationship between C-sections and higher rates of type 1 diabetes and asthma.[92,93,94,95]

Additionally, C-section deliveries have been found to slow one form of the ability of a baby to concentrate—spatial attention—when compared with babies that had experienced vaginal deliveries.[96]

A Resource for Making Choices

The importance of communicating openly with doctors, of asking the right questions for any treatment or procedure, cannot be overstated. Fewer than half of all patients receive clear information on the benefits and tradeoffs of treatments for their conditions.[97,98,99]

A good resource, Choosing Wisely (www.choosingwisely.org) was created to help people learn more about tests and treatments that might be best for them, and which ones, including surgery, might be unnecessary. The website was created with the help of the American Board of Internal Medicine Foundation, a group of medical specialists that works with national organizations to inform the public about health care choices.

Patients and physicians alike can use this website to determine the best approach to specific health issues, and both often use the information to open an informative discussion on the patient's health needs.

Along the way, it's important to place less emphasis on isolated lab numbers or image results and take a closer look at the patient as a whole. It's one of the biggest challenges in the field of health care.

The United States was recently ranked as spending the most money per person on health care worldwide, yet it is ranked 46th worldwide in health care efficiency.[100,101]

If the cost of eggs in the United States rose the way health care costs have risen since 1945, the price of a dozen eggs would now be $55![102] We are spending more and more money on drugs and health care, yet health care quality is not improving in equal measure.

Our health care model, as it is set up, reflects our society and is a mirror that reflects how we view ourselves and our bodies. In other words, culture drives structure. We will benefit as a whole if we make a change in how our society views health care. However, while that process is slowly taking place, this book will help you to take big steps now to achieving better health.

Let's start by looking at another way of viewing our bodies and seeing what nature has to teach us about our health.

What You Can Do Now

- As your body changes, remember that your prescriptions may need to be adjusted accordingly.
- One good source of information on how your prescriptions may be affecting you, especially if you are taking more than one drug, is your pharmacist. He or she has received extensive education on the dynamics of drugs that most MDs haven't. Many MDs don't have the time during your visit to look at all the cross-reactions that can occur with multiple prescriptions. They are under pressure to see a number of patients per hour. Bring your list of meds to your pharmacist to review to make sure that they are not at cross-purposes with each other, or that may be as-

sociated with other symptoms that you are having. Talk to your prescribing doctor if red flags come up.

- The University of Maryland Medical Center has very good Internet resources to look up drug interactions and other information on prescription medicine. Go to http://www.umm.edu, and on the Health Information tab, choose the Drug Interactions Tool.

- The Food and Drug Administration has a Medication Guides section for consumers. It contains information on more than 400 commonly used prescriptions, including what you need to know and what the drug does.[103] Go to fda.gov for more information or to the "Notes" section for a more specific link.

- If you are going to be using prescriptions, discuss with your physician what the signs and symptoms you are experiencing may be telling you about what else is not working well in your body.

- Medical treatment is not always uniform for a particular condition. Choosingwisely.org is a good tool where you can find out whether experts in the field think that a particular test or treatment suggested to you is likely the best one. Consider talking to your doctor if you see discrepancies, or get the proverbial second opinion. Remember that when doctors refer you to health centers where they benefit financially, there is a strong tendency to recommend a lot more tests and surgeries than if they didn't have financial ties to the centers.

- A lot of my patients tell me that the second-opinion doctor is not covered by their insurance plan, especially with HMOs. My usual advice is to tell them to get copies of their files, including lab and imaging results, and pay a board-certified doctor in that specialty for a consultation. You will pay it out of pocket, but it's usually for one visit and usually well worth it, if only for more peace of mind that your treatment plan is the best one for you.

[3]

Can't Stomach It?

LET'S SEE HOW this new way of looking at how our body works can help us with stomachaches. Unfortunately, our culture typically thinks of the human body as a machine, and medical treatment systems mirror this viewpoint of society. Patients are usually treated as if their body were made up of largely isolated parts. That approach leads to taking a pill for this and a pill for that.

When someone develops a symptom, the habitual assumption is that some part of his or her machine is not working properly. So the patient is given a pill that's meant to regulate that body part to make it work either faster or slower.

One example of this is a condition that most of us have had: heartburn. Usually when you go to the doctor's office for this, you are given a prescription or told to take antacids.

There are, however, other reasons why you could be suffering from this; you shouldn't assume that excess acid produced by the stomach is always the cause.

Heartburn can result from one or more systems of your body not functioning properly. In fact, the symptoms, which most assume occur due to too much stomach acid, often occur due to the stomach not producing enough acid.

There might be a reluctance to eat meat, burping after meals, and feeling bloated for a few hours after eating. If these symptoms start to show up half an hour or more after a meal, the gallbladder, not the stomach, might be the issue, especially if foods containing fat or oils are involved.

Unfortunately, the symptoms of having too much or not enough stomach acid can be the same, so it's not always easy to tell them apart.

As we get older, our stomach produces less, not more, stomach acid.[1,2,3,4] The right levels are important for digestive and immune functions. High acidity levels in your stomach, produced by hydrochloric acid, are needed to protect you from bugs and help digesting enzymes work better. These enzymes can be deactivated if the acid levels are too low.

Antacid Alert

However, many people take antacids for heartburn despite having low-stomach-acid issues. In fact, more than 100 million prescriptions are filled each year for stomach acid–suppressing drugs.

These drugs have their place, but often they can create more problems.[5,6] If you take something that lowers your already-low stomach acid levels, such as a proton pump inhibitor, it can impair some of the stomach's other duties, such as helping to kill bacteria. It can also increase the frequency of intestinal bacterial infections and increase the risk of pneumonia.[7]

The government has issued a warning concerning the use of this type of antacid medicine, because low stomach acid levels allow more of these harmful types of bacteria to live, which can also lead to diarrhea.[8,9] Long-term use of these products can be harmful, and it's best to thoroughly discuss their long-term side effects with your physician.

The next time you see a commercial for over-the-counter antacids, hit the record button on your remote. When you play back the commercial, carefully read the fine print that fleetingly shows up, or listen to the quickly spoken warnings at the end that commonly warn against using certain types of medications such as these for more than 14 days without supervision.

Antacids can also increase your risk for food allergies[10] and can affect your body's ability to break down and absorb minerals such as iron, calcium, and magnesium, as well as certain vitamins. This is harmful for a number of reasons; for example, iron-deficiency anemia can be caused by problems with digestion in the stomach.[11,12,13] We will discuss how the effects of these can affect the function of your brain as well.

When you eat foods that require the production of a certain amount of hydrochloric acid in your stomach, such as meats and fish, your stomach might not be able to make enough acid. This can lead to digestive problems, even when you feel that you have produced excess acid and experience that yucky acid feeling creeping up your throat.

A Paradoxical Phenomenon

When your stomach acid is too low, certain foods, such as meats and fish, are not broken down properly during digestion. When this happens, the food begins decomposing in a way that can release organic acids. So the acid you feel creeping up your throat may not be from excess stomach acid—rather, it could be a problem of not producing enough acid.

Another thing to consider is that when you have low stomach acid levels, the food you've eaten moves more quickly through your stomach. The acid helps to digest this food and also acts as a sentry against bacteria and other pathogens. So when food moves faster than normal through your stomach, the stomach acid has less time to protect you from bugs or to prepare your body for better digestion.

On the other hand, people with high levels of stomach acid have a much slower transit time for the food to leave the stomach. It's one of the reasons why they may feel full a few hours after they eat, even very little food, or aren't hungry at all.

In cases where there's too much hydrochloric acid production in the stomach, which is less common than you might think, taking antacids for a short period of time will be helpful for symptom relief.

What else could you consider taking instead of proton pump inhibitors if you suffer from too much stomach acid? Natural ingredients that have helped many include eating okra to start a meal. If the taste does not appeal to you, supplements with okra can be purchased at your local health food store. Another natural product that has worked well for many with heartburn and acid reflux is bentonite clay.

I mentioned that the symptoms of excess stomach acid and insufficient stomach acid often feel the same. So which one is it for you, if you suffer these symptoms?

Here is one way that you can use to give you, and your doctor, a clinical clue. Start by using supplements such as betaine hydrochloric acid with your meal. That is, in effect, the acid that your stomach produces. If this supplement makes your symptoms worse, such as increasing heartburn, it points to your stomach producing too much acid. You may be better off first trying one of the natural supplements I mentioned, such as okra or bentonite clay, or both together.

If, on the other hand, you feel less burn in your stomach after meals, can digest better, and have less burping and smelly gas, it strongly points to low stomach acid issues. Be aware that if you have ulcers, regardless of the level of stomach acid you produce, this supplement may cause you stomachaches. It should not be used in these cases. In all instances, regarding these and other health issues, and I won't repeat this often since it was mentioned in the beginning of the book, check with your doctor for exceptions and contraindications.

Whether you produce too much or not enough stomach acid, you still want to look at why that's happening—to seek out the root causes. Ask yourself, why are my body's self-regulating and healing abilities compromised? Or, what connections am I missing? Look for and address those causes, while giving appropriate relief as your body begins to heal.

Could one of those causes be in your head?

Appropriate levels of secretion of digestive enzymes such as hydrochloric acid, as well as the digestive enzyme associated with it, pepsin, which helps to break down protein in the stomach, can be a result of your brain not functioning properly. Your entire digestive tract can be malfunctioning due to brain issues.

Many times people are prescribed an antacid medication for heartburn or they might be taking natural supplements to help with digestion for years, yet the cause might stem from areas of the brain that are not regulating digestive function properly. As a result, the symptom is a consequence, yet its root causes are not being addressed.

Your Stomach and Brain Atrophy

If you are 60 or over, there are important connections between the health of your stomach and the size of your brain that you need to become aware of. These important connections can have an effect on increasing the risks of developing mild cognitive impairment and Alzheimer's disease.

Around the age of 60, our brain starts to atrophy, or shrink in size. If you know about these connections and take action, there may be simple steps you can take to slow down the rate of atrophy, as well as to give yourself a better opportunity of having a healthier brain, with good memory and concentration.

Good stomach function is one such connection.

As we age, the absorption of nutrients undergoes a decline. Additionally, as I mentioned earlier, as we age, we create less stomach acid. Proper levels of stomach acidity are needed, however, for our stomach to secrete what is known as *intrinsic factor,* which helps our bodies to absorb vitamin B12 in the small intestine.

Low levels of intrinsic factor decrease our ability to absorb this important vitamin. Low levels of B12, along with low levels of folate and vitamin B6, hinder our body's ability to lower the concentration of a substance known as *homocysteine,* which causes brain gray-matter loss.

Higher levels of these vitamins, however, decrease homocysteine and slow brain atrophy in elderly people with mild cognitive impairment who have high homocysteine levels.

That's important, because accelerated brain atrophy is seen in people who progress from mild cognitive impairment to Alzheimer's. High homocysteine levels lead to gray-matter destruction in the medial temporal lobe, the part of the brain associated with memory and Alzheimer's.[14]

Those at risk for Alzheimer's with high homocysteine levels should consider blood testing to determine these vitamin levels. When needed, starting a vitamin B therapy can decrease gray-matter atrophy, or brain loss, in this important area by a factor of seven.[15] Vitamin B12 levels in the blood can vary in a short amount of time. As a result, another test that indicates B12 levels, called a methylmalonic acid test, is usually run. However, this test is not routinely recommended for the elderly because it does not reflect B12 deficiency as well at an advanced age.

Metformin, the most commonly prescribed drug for diabetes, has been shown to markedly lower vitamin B12 levels after years of use.

Later on, I will discuss benefits of chewing foods properly that people aren't usually aware of. One of them has to do with B12. Chewing helps the salivary glands to produce saliva, which binds to this important vitamin in a way that helps the B12 to survive passage through the acidic stomach, which would otherwise break it down, until it gets to the small intestine.

Aids to Digestion

Digestive aids contain an acid that the stomach should produce in normal quantities. Often, patients with this type of acid complaint feel immediate relief, reporting much better digestion, with no burping after meals or reflux. Betaine hydrochloride and pepsin, along with the herb peppermint, can help. Deglycyrrhizinated licorice helps with gastric disorders, including ulcers.

Good calcium absorption is necessary for maintaining healthy bones and other processes. Proper production of stomach secretions is important for good digestion and to help food to be absorbed in your intestines. The stomach helps your intestines to stay healthy.

Small doses of calcium also help to stimulate stomach acid production and can be taken before meals.[16,17,18] You might consider trying gentian, a bitter root that is an excellent digestive aid. In the past few decades, our diets have unfortunately shifted toward sweeter foods.

Many bitter roots and herbs do more than just help the digestive system. They also aid our nervous, cardiovascular, and immune systems.[19,20,21,22,23,24] Many diseases, such as arthritis, diabetes, Alzheimer's, osteoporosis, and heart disease, often start with the same type of cellular changes.

These changes can be mediated by the use of herbs and spices that are bitter to our palate. They act to help slow or stop the progression of many diseases and bring a greater level of health before people are diagnosed with an illness.[25,26,27,28]

I mentioned in the first chapter some of the challenges with correctly diagnosing urinary tract infections (UTIs) and the issue of antibiotic-resistant uropathogens that has arisen. These are the organisms, usually bacteria, that cause UTIs. I noted that there has been research showing that most of the bacteria involved are antibiotic-resistant, and that an herb has been found that is effective against most of these bacteria when antibiotics are not. It's an herb so common that you probably may have eaten some this week: garlic.[29]

A crude water-based extract of garlic has been effective in lab testing in killing 82 percent of the uropathogens that antibiotics could not. Garlic has also been shown to be of help in killing fungi, viruses, and protozoa. More testing will take place to find out more on bioavailability and other dynamics. Meanwhile, ask your doctor to consider garlic as a nutritional adjunct to his or her treatment plan.[30]

There can be many reasons why someone may be having issues with producing the proper amount of stomach acid. An individual can have more than one obstacle to the body's being able to regulate it. The clinician not only must always get a sense for what will eliminate the symptom but also should be attentive to connections within the body that can cause or prolong the problem.

For example, the stomach lining does a lot of its regeneration during sleep,[31,32] so sleeping disorders can contribute to stomach issues and digestive disorders.

Other conditions can affect the stomach, such as autoimmune disorders, hernias involving the stomach, bacterial infections, cancer, anemia, nutritional deficiencies, brain dysfunction, genetics, and emotions.

In most chronic diseases, there is usually more than one reason why the body is not able to heal itself.

With that in mind, let's take a closer look at how your body is connected in ways that help heal you . . . or cause more problems.

What You Can Do Now

- Consider bitters and herbal aids to help with digestive issues.
- For those over 60 who have mild cognitive impairment and digestive issues, consider homocysteine blood testing to see if vitamin and cofactors therapy is needed to help with the health of the brain.
- When in doubt . . . chew.

[4]

Exploring Your Body's Connections

MANY PEOPLE WOULD be surprised at just how important is the role that the rest of their body plays in helping to heal conditions and illnesses they may have.

For example, did you know that your bones help your pancreas and your body's insulin receptors to work better? These seemingly disparate processes are indeed connected, and knowing about them will help us to understand how a healthy body really works and what we can do about promoting health.

Let's explore another connection that at first glance is not apparent. That's the connection between depression and digestion. Increasing the number of beneficial bacteria in your gut has been shown to be helpful with depression. Having a healthy gut can help your brain to work better.[1,2,3]

There is also some evidence pointing to a surprising connection between the gut and Parkinson's disease, indicating that the disease may have its origin in the gastrointestinal tract and reach the brain through the *vagus* nerve, a nerve prominent in digestive functions.[4]

Ingesting beneficial bacteria like those found in fermented foods has also been shown to help decrease high blood pressure and cholesterol. Doing so helps keep the bad bacteria and other organisms in check, whereas the wrong types of gut microbes can stimulate colon cancer growth.[5,6,7,8]

Fermented foods contain vitamin K, which helps optimize vascular and bone health.[9,10,11] Additionally, vitamin K, particularly K2, which is converted as well as produced by healthy bacteria in the gut, not only helps with osteoporosis but also aids the body in handling sugar. Further, vitamin K2 aids in the production of *osteocalcin,* which helps strengthen bone, stimulate insulin production, and improve insulin sensitivity.[12,13,14]

Sauerkraut, anyone?

If sauerkraut isn't your cup of green tea, another option is yogurt. Exercise care, since many of the store-bought yogurts have sugar added. Additionally, a number of commercial yogurts might not have many live bacteria left by the time you eat them.

Supplements are also a quick way of getting beneficial gut bacteria, but whole foods are always best. Miso soup, soy sauce, kefir, sauerkraut, and pickles are some good examples.

Green leafy foods, as well as dairy products, have lots of vitamin K. There are various types of vitamin K. All have important functions. The ones found in the foods mentioned above are type K1. Gut bacteria transforms K1 into K2, which also helps your body to work better.

However, even if you eat a cow's daily portion of greens, if you have a malfunctioning gut and don't have good amounts of healthy gut bugs, they won't be able to metabolize the type of vitamin K in the food to the one that you need.

People with intestinal dysfunctions, or who use antacids, aspirin, or antibiotics frequently, may be at risk for low levels of vitamin K2.

Connections, anyone, between the heart, achy joints, and gut bacteria?

Let's look at what can happen if you have digestive issues as it relates to vitamin K2. Gut issues can lead to low levels of vitamin K2; low vitamin K2 is associated with higher cardiovascular risks. Since K2 helps calcium to be deposited in the skeleton and not the joints in your body, it can not only help to make your bones stronger, but also help to keep calcific deposits associated with osteoarthritis out of your joints.

Health Connections

Now, on to more health connections that are important but not obvious.

For example, could there be a connection between depression and a disease that people associate with the ovaries? Women diagnosed with *polycystic ovary syndrome* (PCOS) have higher levels of depression than healthy women.

Up to 10 percent of women of childbearing age have PCOS, many of them without knowing it. Women with PCOS are also more likely to be hospitalized; be diagnosed with diabetes; and have higher levels of stress, anxiety, and miscarriages.[15]

It is not necessary to have ovarian cysts—or, to be more precise, ovarian follicles, in order to be diagnosed with PCOS. In fact, most women with PCOS do not have ovarian cysts.[16]

Interestingly enough, men can genetically carry PCOS, often manifesting as premature baldness. PCOS seems to have a genetic component and is associated with hormone imbalance, and often with insulin resistance, high blood pressure, and increased weight. For those with PCOS and weight issues, losing even a modest amount of weight can help to bring hormones more in balance.

Throughout this book, we will be discussing a number of things that you need to be aware of to help your body to heal, as well as emphasizing underlying barriers to healing. These barriers can range from internal dysfunctions that don't permit our body's systems to self-regulate, to environmental challenges. That's important, because helping to facilitate your body's innate ability to recuperate at all levels leads to deeper healing.

You can experience a number of symptoms elsewhere in the body that you would not typically make a connection to being brain-related. These include digestive issues that go beyond digestive enzyme production.

Areas of the brain depend on other areas of the body in order to work well. They help coordinate the function of other areas, working in intricate, connected networks.

Let's suppose someone is suffering from depression, memory loss, and fatigue, which are usually symptoms of a brain that is not working properly, or from brain degeneration (since brain cells are called *neurons,* the clinical term for this is *neuronal degeneration*).

Several issues can account for these symptoms, but digestive issues are frequently associated with brain dysfunction—or brain fatigue, to use a common phrase. Issues that can contribute to this condition include poor brain circulation, decreased oxygen supply, decreased stable fuel for the brain in the form of glucose, gut and brain inflammation, thyroid issues, trauma, and anemia.

Parts of the brain work together to coordinate functions, but the back of the brain, known as the *hindbrain,* is the part more directly responsible for helping with digestion.

Let's look at someone who is complaining of digestive issues and also has difficulty concentrating, reasoning, and planning; feels depressed; and has lost the motivation to remain active.

These could be signs that the front of the brain, the *frontal cortex,* is not working well. When the frontal cortex is not working properly, the ability to modulate how a part of the midbrain works can be affected.

When the front of our brain, the part that we use to make plans and reasoned decisions, is not working well, it can create an imbalance of nerve activation between the "fight or flight" part of our nervous system, known as the *sympathetic nervous system,* and the "rest and digest" part of our nervous system, known as the *parasympathetic nervous system.*

The effect is that the excitable sympathetic nervous system usually works at stronger levels, while the restful, digestive parasympathetic nervous system might not be. If parts of the brain are not working well, they might not activate other parts of the brain associated with digestion as well as they should. The enteric nervous system, which is also involved with digestion, is similarly affected.

Decreased involvement of these important brain centers that regulate digestion can also affect gallbladder contractions, which can lead to gallstone formations. And when these rest-and-digest vagal centers of your brain are not firing as they should, the valves in your intestines might not work as well as they should.

The effects of this brain dysfunction can alter the way the muscles in your intestines move the food through them and move waste products out of the body, causing constipation. Further, brain dysfunction has been shown to be a central process leading to irritable bowel syndrome.[17]

Illustrating the strength of this connection between gut and brain health, a study found that intestinal damage could be observed as soon as three hours after a brain injury occurred.[18] A similar study revealed that a number of patients with inflammatory bowel disease had the same brain lesions as patients with multiple sclerosis—and nearly as frequently.[19]

This drives an important point home: treating digestive issues is not just about providing natural supplements or prescription drugs for your digestive tract. It's important to work on all associated issues so that every part of your body, including your brain, functions as part of a healing network.

When healing does not happen, symptoms that are a consequence of dysfunction appear. And they can stay for long periods of time—often for many years. During that time, they can change in intensity or come and go.

Unfortunately, most clinical approaches focus primarily on prescribing drugs that are chemically effective at suppressing symptoms. They have an important but limited value. The function of drugs is typically to force the body to do something or to suppress function. Unfortunately, not enough time is usually spent looking for subtler, interconnected causative factors, including connections that could help you to resolve underlying issues that are not allowing your body to heal fully.

Osteoporosis: Hidden Connections

Let's take osteoporosis as an example of hidden connections within your body that may help, or hinder, your effort to have healthy bones. It's a complex subject involving a number of factors, many outside the scope of this book.

Most know that lower estrogen levels, particularly during the first few years before and after menopause, can weaken bones. There are other connections, however, that are also important to know about. Progesterone levels also begin to decrease a few years before menopause, leading to a thinning of bone. Thyroid dysfunction, kidney issues, problems with your adrenal glands, and rheumatoid arthritis can also lead to osteoporosis.

When men undergo a decrease in testosterone, it can also end up leading to bone loss. Men metabolize varying amounts of testosterone into estrogen.

Other hormones that can affect bone health include *didehydroepiandrosterone,* commonly known as DHEA; *follicle stimulating hormone,* which also helps with the function of sexual organs; and *cortisol.* Your doctor can help to make sure that the levels of these hormones are appropriate for strong bones. Doing so can help to keep you further away from hip or other types of fractures in your golden years.

Ever wonder where the bone loss ends up? As your bone mineral density decreases, your bone is broken down into metabolites. One of them is *deoxypyridinoline,* which is released through your urine.

It's important to know that a simple urine test to measure bone metabolite loss can give you and your doctor an idea of what your rate of bone loss is, and whether the therapies being used are helpful. DEXA scans and other tests for bone density give you a snapshot of where you are over the months and years;

however, this type of urine test can give an indication of what is occurring metabolically with bone loss now, and can guide treatment.

Clinical testing for the hormones that I mentioned before can also be of help to monitor appropriate levels, since they are important for the health of your bones.

Patients with osteoporosis are usually given one of two types of medication. One type stimulates the bones to increase bone formation, and the other type is prescribed to slow bone loss, or a combination of both. There are a number of factors that come into play to help your body to produce bone naturally, one of which involves the liver. It is important for your liver to function in a way that produces an amino acid called *taurine*, which has been found to be important for bone formation.[20]

The liver has to work well to help avoid osteoporosis. However, the clinical picture is more complex than that. We've talked about how your stomach needs to work well enough to help your body to absorb calcium, which is necessary for bone health, right?

Well, your stomach also has to be healthy enough, by producing intrinsic factor, to help you absorb vitamin B12 in your small intestine, which stimulate the liver to make what it needs for you to have stronger bones.[21]

An emphasis on calcium intake and vitamin D for the prevention and treatment of osteoporosis is well established. There are, however, other connections between healthy bones and food that many people aren't aware of.

Our modern lifestyle finds us eating an increasing number of acidic-type foods, such as animal products, most grains, refined cereals, junk food, and most prescription drugs.

What's the big deal with high levels of acid? you might ask. High acidity in the body leads to bone loss and loss of lean body mass.[22]

The amount of base minerals we ingest that counteract acidity has decreased, to the detriment of our overall health, including our bone health. Base minerals include minerals such as potassium, magnesium, and calcium. They are alkaline and therefore help to balance the acid levels produced by eating other types of foods. The resultant pH levels, which measure the net interaction between both types, can be tested in our blood and urine. A multimineral supplementation significantly increases blood and urinary pH, which is generally a good thing for the health of our bones and our bodies.[23]

Among the base minerals, potassium is particularly important.

Potassium is commonly found in fruits and vegetables. It can help you to reduce your dietary acid load, reduce your blood pressure, increase the amount of muscle mass in your body, improve the health of your blood vessels, reduce the risk of stroke, and, yes, decrease bone loss! Americans, however, eat around half of the amount recommended. Back in the Stone Age, our ancestors were eating over four times as much as we do.[24] Unfortunately, what we eat a lot more of now is . . . sodium, as in table salt. In fact, we eat over seven times more sodium than potassium, compared with our cave-dwelling troglodytes! That's a lot of stress on our kidneys and can have a detrimental effect on blood pressure levels.

A point made throughout this book is that most of our health issues are multifactorial—that a this-for-that approach does not meet all of our needs to heal at the deepest levels. This also includes something as straightforward as ingesting potassium. There are foods that have good potassium levels but are acidic in nature, such as some cereals, meat, and milk products.

You need not only potassium but also bicarbonate precursors to reduce the acid load in your body. Those are usually found in fruits and vegetables.

Higher potassium intake, which helps to drive down the acid levels in the body, is associated with a reduction of stroke risk.[25,26] Lower potassium levels in the elderly are associated with increased risk of stroke.[27] In a study involving more than 5,000 people, those taking diuretics had low potassium levels and were at greater risk for stroke.[28] Some people have health conditions that warrant low potassium diets and should consult with their prescribing physician if they want to find out more.

Of the many natural sources for better bone health, one that most people would not associate with stronger bones is a protein that is produced by many glands in our bodies, *lactoferrin*.

It is an iron-binding protein present in milk, colostrum, whey protein, the mammary gland, and other glands in our body. Not only can it help to build strong bones, but also it serves to boost our immune response, protects against neurodegenerative diseases,[29] and is antimicrobial.[30] Lactoferrin has potential benefits in the treatment of breast, colon, and other types of cancer;[31,32,33] can increase iron levels in pregnant women and children;[34] and can decrease inflammation. It has also been shown to be effective against intestinal toxins[35] and *H. pylori* infections.[36]

Those who have intolerance to milk may find that highly purified lactoferrin supplements may not be a problem, since the protein composition in lactorferrin is different from that in lactose, the milk sugar. Lactoferrin does not contain lactose. For those who have issues with the proteins in milk that usually lead to allergic reactions (bovine serum albumin, lactalbumin, casein and its derivatives, beta-lactoglobulin), those proteins are not found in lactoferrin.

Let's put our attention on lactoferrin's effects on bone growth. I mentioned earlier that many osteoporosis drugs work by stimulating bone growth, which is done by cells in our bodies known as *osteoblasts*, or by the breakdown of bone, accomplished via cells known as *osteoclasts*.

Lactoferrin increases bone building naturally. Animal studies show that it stimulates osteoblastic, or bone growth, activity, and decreases the activity of the osteoclasts, which reduces the bone matrix.[37,38,39,40] Researchers have described it as a "potent regulator of bone cell activity."[41] More studies on its promising bone-building effects for humans are under way.

The human body is truly the most wonderful, complicated construct in the universe. The more we are able to be aware of and engage with the intricate connectedness within our body, the greater our chances for healing.

Speaking of connectedness, let's continue to explore at a deeper level the connection between depression and digestion.

Depression and Digestion

Neurotransmitters are chemical messengers, and when one of these messengers—for example, *serotonin*—is low, then depression is thought to set in. This happens when the brain is not functioning well. One type of antidepressant drug commonly prescribed for this—SSRIs, or *selective serotonin reuptake inhibitors*—is designed to keep your serotonin levels high to decrease depression.

However, the long-standing belief that depression is due to low serotonin levels, and the long-term usefulness of SSRI drug types for depression, are being questioned as a result of new research.

It seems that people might have higher, rather than lower, levels of serotonin in their brain during episodes of depression. Recent research points in an interesting direction—namely, that the decreases of serotonin seen in a clinically significant number of patients on SSRIs are due to the body fighting the effects of the drug. The authors of this study think that this type of drug can, in the long term, make it harder to recover from depression.[42]

Another study links high, rather than low, serotonin levels in mice with greater levels of anxiety. The research on depression and serotonin levels is indicating that the issue is not as simple as determining the level of serotonin. Instead, it appears that how serotonin is chemically bonded has an effect on the brain's internal environment.[43,44,45] More research will shed further light on hidden connections between this neurotransmitter and your emotions.

There are a number of natural aids to also consider for depression. Something as simple as exercise can be helpful, along with herbs such as kava[46] and St. John's wort, fish oil, and B vitamins. For example, folate, a type of B vitamin, can help reduce depression. If you have a folate deficiency, it can also affect how well you respond to antidepressants that involve increasing serotonin production levels.[47]

Microcurrent stimulation has been shown to help reduce depression, as well as anxiety and insomnia.[48,49,50,51,52,53]

The therapeutic use of pulsed light, involving audiovisual brainwave synchronization, which is therapy that uses light and sound, has been shown to have an effect on neurotransmitter levels. It has also been shown to be effective in alleviating depression, memory and concentration issues, seasonal affective disorder, and attention deficit disorder.[54,55,56,57,58,59,60,61]

The application of healing approaches involving light and sound can have powerful effects on our health.

Intestinal inflammation is associated with a low amount of beneficial bacteria in the gut, and gut inflammation releases chemicals that can create brain inflammation. Research shows that children with more frequent stomachaches usually have higher levels of depression when they become adults, revealing another important connection between gut dysfunction and brain dysfunction.[62,63,64]

Let's look at more connections between your gut, what you eat, and your health.

Emulsifiers, which are found in most processed foods, can change the composition of the bacteria in your gut, leading to gut inflammation and metabolic syndrome.[65] On the other hand, having a diverse and well-balanced amount of bacteria in the gut can prevent issues with metabolic syndrome, which about 35 percent of adults have.

Gluten Sensitivity: What You Can Do about It

A growing number of children and adults complain of stomachaches because they might be sensitive to foods that contain gluten. This protein is found in products containing wheat, rye, and barley, but oats can be contaminated with gluten from those grains as well. Gluten is used in baking to make bread chewy and to help it rise in the oven.

In the past 50 years or so, the occurrence of gluten sensitivity, the most extreme form of which is celiac disease, has increased. The symptoms associated with this issue include depression, skin rashes, nausea, bloating, and anemia, among others. There has been a sharp increase in the number of people diagnosed with celiac disease, yet better detection is not the reason.

This increase has coincided with the introduction of genetically changed strains of grains, particularly wheat. That, above all other factors, seems to be the reason that accounts for more patients having this problem.[66,67]

Some people who have issues with gluten might find that they can tolerate eating bread and other products again by using organic, primitive grains that have not been genetically altered. In research involving patients with celiac disease, biopsies revealed that eating these older grain types did not cause the usual intestinal cell inflammation and immune responses associated with the disease.[68,69,70,71,72] You can look for "heritage grains" on the Internet for more information.

Most people suffering from gluten sensitivity don't complain of problems with their intestines and aren't aware that there might be a connection. That's because often seemingly unrelated symptoms are usually the issue and usually involve the brain. The connection is so strong that a number of neurologists view gluten sensitivity as primarily a neurological disease.[73]

What about our genes and their role in bowel issues? Much has been written in the media about genetic testing for digestive challenges that include *single nucleotide polymorphisms* (SNPs). Popular tests are available through the mail that give users and their genetic counselors useful information about their genetic profile and how it may affect how well some systems in their body may function.

Beyond SNPs and their effect on the expression of genes are other types of important genetic dynamics, such as structural variants known as *copy number variations* (CNVs). An SNP involves one nucleotide base. A CNV can involve thousands to millions of nucleotide bases. It is estimated that up to 25 percent of our genes may have CNVs.

What's a CNV? In simple terms, think of your genes as a piece of paper with a string of typed letters on it being duplicated by a copy machine. But the copies come out differently than the original. Sometimes the copy is missing some letters, sometimes the order of the letters is changed, or sometimes there are extra letters.

Every time you make a copy that does not have the letters exactly as were typed on the original piece of paper, you have created a CNV. Your body produces a certain amount of these copies, and that number can vary from one part of the body to another. It can also vary from country to country.[74] In chapter 22, I will discuss research showing how the number of CNVs associated with an aspect of your digestion can have up to an eightfold effect on your weight!

Now, on to what CNVs have to do with digestive issues. People with fewer than four CNVs for antimicrobial cells in the intestines will have greater inflammation in the gut and a greater susceptibility to Crohn's disease.[75]

You may think at this point, "Great, give me lots of those same CNVs." However, as I've noted, simple addition or subtraction dynamics rarely gives us deeper glimpses into how our bodies really respond. For example, if the number of copies is greater than four for these *beta-defensin genes*, as they are known, then any minor injury to your skin can result in a strong inflammatory response and a greater risk of psoriasis.[76]

These are just a couple of examples of the effect on our health of CNVs. As you can see, our body's complexity precludes us from assuming that even genetic therapy should have only one primary focus, whether SNPs, CNVs, or other structural genetic variants.

Let's take a look at another factor that can influence how well your digestive system handles the challenges that a lot of modern foods pose. Consumption of foods that contain pesticides such as *glyphosate*, which is the active ingredient in Roundup, has been linked to gluten intolerance and to disruption of gut bacteria.[77,78,79]

In chapter 22, "Mirror, Mirror," I will discuss how pesticides can make it harder to lose weight and to keep it off.

Imbalances in the gut bacteria, which pesticides contribute to, are connected to decreased brain health. Total pesticide use for 21 major crops in the U.S. increased fivefold between 1961 and 2008.[80] Glyphosate use has increased sharply over the past 15 years. It is the most commonly used pesticide in the U.S., with over 200 million pounds used yearly. Of these, approximately 7 million pounds are applied annually to home yards and gardens.[81]

As you can see, a lot of issues arise from problems with our digestion, and problems elsewhere in our body can cause digestive issues. For example, a healthy gut can affect your mood. Researchers studied several patients' brain activity in an MRI, separating patients who had taken *probiotics*—which increase the beneficial bacteria in the gut—and those who had not. They found that those who had taken probiotics showed a change in activity in the brain regions associated with the central processing of emotions and sensations, including experiencing less anxiety.[82,83]

Imagine going to a psychiatrist, and instead of being asked about your childhood, the doctor asks if you've been eating fermented foods or taking probiotics and how well your digestion has been working!

Clinicians can best serve the needs of their patients by first addressing the underlying issues that hinder the healing process—often before prescribing any medication. At the same time, they can address the symptoms by providing symptomatic relief to the patient.

Let's explore why we receive clinical care in pieces: that is, take one prescription for this problem, another prescription for that other problem, etc., as if the organs and systems of our bodies existed in isolation.

Where does this type of clinical approach come from?

What You Can Do Now

- Among other conditions, ingesting beneficial bacteria like those found in fermented foods has been shown to help decrease high blood pressure, metabolic syndrome, depression, and cholesterol. Fermented foods, especially ones that have not been pasteurized, are valuable sources. Unpasteurized ones include probiotic supplements, live cultured pickled vegetables, sauerkraut, cheese made from raw milk, kimchi, unpasteurized miso (which has not been heated), kombucha tea and fermented drinks, and yogurt and kefir that have been made with live cultures (not all the commercially sold ones are).

Nondairy yogurt varieties can also contain live cultures.

- Gluten-sensitivity issues are also neurological. Some people who have issues with gluten might find that they can tolerate eating bread and other products again by using organic, primitive grains that have not been genetically altered. Look for heritage grains on the Internet.

- For those with polycystic ovary syndrome and weight issues, losing even a modest amount of weight can help to bring hormones more in balance.

- Eating fruits and vegetables will decrease the acidity in our body and increase our potassium levels, which are typically low. Potassium bicarbonate can be bought in health food stores. If you eat like most people do, then four to five grams a day will be a good help to increase your low potassium levels.

- A number of natural aids for depression are available. Something as simple as exercise can be helpful, along with herbs such as kava and St. John's wort, fish oil, folate, and B vitamins. Consult with your clinician.

- The application of therapies involving light and sound, such as audiovisual brainwave synchronization, can help your brain to work better and to change your mood.

[5]

Our Health in Pieces

PATIENTS ARE OFTEN given medication with the expectation that they will be taking it for years, perhaps for the rest of their lives.

That can be necessary in a number of cases, but it's questionable as to how many. Some of these drugs state, on the tiny print on the label or the insert accompanying the bottle, that they're only to be taken for a short period of time. Others have a long list of side effects in the fine print. A number of these side effects can be cumulative.

Ideally, however, doctors would focus more time on helping patients to develop healthier response states, so that the mind and body can better regulate the healing process before issues develop into full-blown illnesses or pathology. Focusing on healthier responses affords the body a better opportunity to resolve emerging conditions on its own.

I believe that this should be the most important long-term goal of any physician and should become the primary goal of our health care system.

However, the way health care is generally approached in this country is a reflection of how our society feels and thinks about health and illness. Once you start thinking beyond the usual boundaries, it becomes easier to gain a new perspective about your health that can help you solve many health challenges.

How did we arrive at our current view of health? Our present-day approach evolved largely from the Industrial Revolution, in the mid- to late 19th century. That's when we witnessed dramatic advances in machines that shifted Western nations from agricultural societies to more industrial-based societies.

These new machines and what they could do fascinated us; at that time, engineers were considered artists. When something was wrong in a structure or a machine, they studied each component to see where the defective part was; then that component was fixed or replaced.

We are still working with a health model that in many ways is more than 150 years old and in strong need of change.

The Industrial Revolution was a time when people were taken in by the spectacle of machines. These machines represented a big change in their lives and in the economy. However, a machine is a closed system. Our bodies, however, are open-ended, interacting continuously in a dynamic way with our internal and external environments. Moreover, you and I don't respond in a mechanical way as machines do. If we did, people wouldn't have such variable responses to the same drug prescription, treatment plan, or surgery.

Treating the body the way a mechanic fixes a car might be helpful at times or for short-term measures, but inadequate to more fully address the complex, dynamic, and interconnected needs that we have.

In the field of psychiatry during that time, the force of this historical mechanical approach was so strong that psychological illnesses were considered to be due to physical malfunctions. The approach to mental issues was largely mechanical—if you could find the physical cause, it was assumed that you could fix the psychological problem.

We haven't transitioned our health care from this older model to a better one that reflects the human body's true health dynamics, one that needs to include the depth of its connectivity.

Try to imagine the time before industrial machines were powering our societies, our streetlights, and our economies. Before the advent of more recent advances in science, which include our wonderful medical technology, physicians worked differently—by necessity.

They worked with the rhythms and cycles of nature, seeking to understand the body from the perspective of nature and helping to heal the body through what was found in nature.

What do you think would happen at a hospital if, in the middle of the day, the electricity went out and there was no backup power supply? How much diagnosing would be done in that situation, without machines plugged into power sources?

Before modern technology and sophisticated machines, even before the first line of antibiotics—sulfa drugs and, later, penicillin—were available, doctors made house calls and relied heavily on all five of their senses. They closely examined everything to find clues as to why their patient's body was not functioning as it should.

One of the first things many of these physicians did when they entered their patient's home was to sniff the air. More often than not, they got an indication of what was going on simply by the smell. To put this into perspective in modern science, animals are now being used to smell for lung cancer, tuberculosis, and other diseases.[1,2,3,4,5]

Physicians from earlier times also tasted the skin of their patients, because it gave them information about their patients' salt levels and pH. Their tactile senses were highly developed, as was their ability to listen for certain sounds in the body.

We still have those abilities; they just need to be developed, whether it is a physician listening to the sounds of the body or something more exotic, like traditional "fish listeners" from Malaysia, who distinguish the sounds made by different types of fish from long distances simply by putting their head in the water and listening. Contrast that with a recent study involving over 1,000 cardiologists. The large majority of them who took an auscultation test to see if they could detect basic heart murmurs were unable to do so more than half the time. The researchers attributed this to declining auscultatory skills.[6]

If we look at this in terms of applying it to ourselves in everyday life, mothers who kiss their children and discover that the skin usually tastes salty would be interested to know that it could indicate the possibility that their child may have cystic fibrosis.[7,8]

Early physicians paid attention to everything, in large part because they had no other choice. They created a treatment plan for their patients' benefit that was based on all their insights, including observing and examining the condition of their patients by using only their five senses.

To best handle our health challenges, physicians would find advantage in placing less emphasis on isolated lab or image results and taking a closer view of the patient as a whole. It's one of the biggest challenges in the health field: to examine each person as a whole and use technology judiciously.

The patients' best role is to be mindful of connections between how they live their life and what their body might be telling them through their symptoms.

In fact, another way of defining symptoms is that they are your body's way of telling you something needs to change. Keep in mind that where you are experiencing the symptom can be in a different area than where the cause is.

A clear example is a severely obese person developing knee or hip problems. You treat the damaged joints but also focus on reducing the cause, the excess weight. When I ask some female patients if their headaches become more frequent before their periods, looking at how the body is handling hormone clearance can be helpful. Skin issues can be associated with stress on the liver, even in the absence of red flags on the blood tests. We have discussed the connection between low iron and poor stomach function.

Sometimes symptom presentations are such that they need to involve a doctor; other times there are connections that you can make to get better on your own. The purpose of this book is to help you to make these connections and to improve your health, and life, whether or not you require clinical assistance.

No single health discipline has all the answers, however; practitioners of all health disciplines help their patients best by proverbially joining hands and working together.

Next, let's take at look how the connections between seemingly unrelated things, like new farming practices and traffic lights, can help you to see your health differently, and improve it.

What You Can Do Now

- Symptoms are your body's way of saying that something else is not working well. That something else, perhaps more than one thing, needs your attention—the root cause.

- Ask yourself what you can do to help your body better regulate its own healing processes, instead of simply looking to take something, even if it is a natural supplement, to make a symptom go away. Do a mental checklist. The basics are food, water, exercise, and how you are handling your life's stress patterns. Choose the easiest daily habit you think you can change or just stop doing, and try that for a start. After a month, once the change has become second nature, choose the next-easiest habit that you know is not good for you, and drop that one for a month.
- Then, the month after that . . .

[6]

What Color Is Your Traffic Light?

I MADE A reference earlier about underlying barriers to healing. Since I've used the analogy of a garden, let's continue with that.

Let's take the example of a farmer who has been tilling his fields for generations, just like his father and grandfather before him.

With today's challenges of drought, soil erosion, nitrogen runoff, and other environmental issues at play, he considers changing his approach to one that is based more on how nature works and heals. What if he were to put down his plow and choose to work more with nature, using cover crops, green manures, and other soil-enhancing methods?

How well would he do with this approach? Would his fields flourish?

Well, according to research, it's already happening, and with striking results. No-till farming, where the farmer works more closely with nature and its cycles and does not till the soil, is increasing the productivity of crops, decreasing water evaporation and soil erosion. It also decreases nitrogen runoff, which is an environmental hazard.[1]

This important paradigm shift in farming, in changing our viewpoint about how to work with nature, has important parallels with how we can best care for our garden of health.

Good soil, as we know, needs many components—physical, chemical, and biological. Some would include electromagnetic and energetic dynamics.

It's the same with our body. A number of components, or body systems, at first blush don't seem to be connected but, in truth, need to work well together in order to sustain a healthier body.

To have good soil, you need all components present and interacting properly. It's the same with your body and your systems of healing. If these components aren't functioning and working to help each other, they can lay the unfortunate foundation for acute or chronic symptoms and diseases.

Many of the chronic health concerns that bring people in to see doctors are a consequence of one or more of these supportive body systems not working well. Patients often end up being medicated in an attempt to reduce these symptoms; however, not enough attention is paid to helping the other organs and systems in the body that can aid our body to heal.

Our Body Systems

According to the World Health Organization, an agency of the United Nations, there are thousands of diseases and illnesses worldwide.[2,3] Yet our body comprises only a few systems—12 in all, depending on how they are grouped:

1. The nervous system—the brain, spinal cord, and nerves
2. The digestive system—the mouth, stomach, and intestines
3. The cardiovascular system—the heart and blood vessels
4. The skeletal system—the bones and connective tissues
5. The muscular system
6. The skin
7. The endocrine system
8. The lymphatic system—it helps the body to handle toxins
9. The respiratory system
10. The immune system
11. The urinary system
12. The reproductive system

One of these 12 systems is known as the *master control system*. That's the nervous system, which consists of the brain, the spinal cord, and the nerves.

These nerves connect to every cell of every organ in your body and do more than just send information back and forth to the brain. They are also a source of nutrients for a number of cells.[4,5,6,7,8,9] The nerves transport growth factors to the muscle cells of your body through a process known as *axoplasmic transport.*[10]

Does the connection between nerves and muscles have anything to do with our health as we get older?

Aging comes from a Greek word that means "experience." As we age, our nerves do not communicate as well with our muscles, contributing to muscle loss.[11,12] Studies also show that a decrease in the percentage of muscle in our body, along with an increased percentage of fat, is associated with declining health.[13,14] Maintaining muscle tone through exercises such as lifting weights becomes more important with each passing decade.

The best way to maintain a fully healthy body is to naturally support each of these systems so that they can function at their best. When patients heed this advice, I am usually happily surprised to often hear that they are feeling relief from symptoms that I wasn't aware they had!

I've noticed that when it comes to considering underlying issues for most patients, the adrenal, sugar-handling, digestive, liver, and/or nervous system functions have to be looked at closely. That includes, but is not limited to, stress-related conditions. I've often seen discrete long-term dysfunction in one or more of these systems that ends up manifesting as symptoms typically associated with other systems or organs, especially for those with chronic problems.

The correlation between an apparently unrelated set of symptoms and these body systems can be subtle. It might not appear clinically, and as I mentioned before, it might not show up on lab work.

What Does My Lab Work Really Mean?

There are differences between pathological, or disease-level, laboratory test ranges and functional lab ranges. For many lab results, you usually have to wait until you are sick enough to the point where you're in the bottom 5 percent of what is broadly considered to be a normal segment of the population before the test result is flagged as abnormal.[15] Usually, insurance companies won't pay for treatment for conditions that do not show up as abnormal on these lab tests.

Patients know, however, that they are not well, despite lab or imaging studies that show nothing is supposedly wrong. Sometimes the lab results look fine when looked at a more subtle functional level, even though the patient is still experiencing a lot of problems and is frustrated when told that nothing is wrong.

Health as a Traffic Light

Another way that you can think of your health status is as a traffic light. That's right, a simple traffic light. What you often see in clinical approaches, including those that use imaging studies and blood tests, is that the patient isn't considered to have anything wrong until his or her red lights are flashing: abnormal lab results or test findings.

However, most people are suffering in what I call the yellow-light zone. They don't feel well, they don't have any energy, they might be feeling depressed, and they know that their body is causing them discomfort. But when they go for a checkup, they are told that nothing is wrong—no red lights!

Since the majority of blood-test results aren't considered abnormal until they are in the bottom 5 percent, that means a lot of patients with below-average health will have blood tests that show up as normal—even though something's obviously not right. The result of a lab test such as one for the most commonly tested thyroid health marker, known as the *TSH* test, can vary by a factor of 10 before it is considered abnormal.

Many patients are told that there is nothing wrong with them on the basis of often extensive blood tests. However, there's a reason why a blood test, or lab test, is not called a "health test"—that term goes beyond the measure of the lab test's isolated parameters. A lot of patients in the yellow-light health zone feel bad and frustrated for years, or even decades, but their lab results are not reflective of their yellow-light health status.

I noted that I often see dysfunctions in how other systems of the body are working that over time can lead to seemingly unrelated symptoms and conditions. Many don't show up on imaging or lab testing. Although it's beyond the scope of this book to go into each one of the body systems in detail, I want to let you know how important it is to work with helping to improve the function of these systems. They help each other.

They are the foundation of good health—your body's equivalent of good, healthy garden soil.

Fat and Skinny?

There's been a lot of emphasis in the media and in doctor visits on losing weight for better health, and rightly so. However, throughout this book I have been pointing out the importance of going beyond the one-dimensional approach to health. This also applies to weight loss.

Some people are considered to be of normal weight or even low-normal weight. We would not think of them as fat. Yet, is it possible to be skinny and fat at the same time?

Yes!

The term for it is *skinny fat*. The traditional way of measuring how well you are doing with your weight is by using a calculation measuring your height and weight called the *body mass index* (BMI). You are considered to be of normal weight, overweight, or obese, depending on your BMI score.

However, this is a narrowly defined way of looking at body weight. Bodybuilders or fit people with a larger-than-average amount of muscle mass are considered overweight by this standard—almost half of NBA players would be considered overweight using BMI values.

On the other hand, people who have a BMI value indicating that they are of normal weight, yet have less muscle mass than optimal and carry more fat than is healthy—usually around the waist—have higher incidences of diabetes and other problems, including cardiometabolic risk factors. Fat around the organs, known as *visceral fat*, is more harmful than fat in other parts of the body.[16] Visceral fat stimulates changes in a type of immune cell known as a *macrophage,* which makes our body more resistant to insulin and leads to hardening of the arteries and to heart issues.

We are seeing the importance of looking beyond any one measure to determine how well we are. Now let's discuss health and vitality from a perspective that's different from what we're used to, and learn more about how our body helps itself to heal at deeper levels.

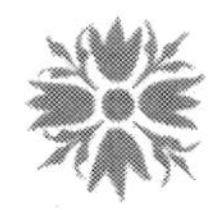

What You Can Do Now

- When considering underlying issues for most people, the adrenal, sugar-handling, digestive, liver, and/or nervous-system functions have to be addressed closely. If they are not working well, other parts of the body will feel the effects over time, and seemingly unrelated symptoms may arise.
- Lab tests that come back negative do not mean you are healthy or even that the systems that the blood test looked at are working optimally. If you get "normal" results and don't feel well, don't be discour-

aged—keep asking questions. Know that testing measures are only limited health parameters.

- Weight is also something to take in context. You want an adequate amount of muscle mass in order to be healthy. Research shows it makes a difference, especially in older people. Fat around the tummy is the worst of all, since it is especially harmful to the rest of your body. If you have love handles, more fat loss may be necessary. Later we will talk about the difference between losing volume versus losing density.

[7]

The Power That Heals You

WHEN WE SPEAK of underlying barriers to healing at a fundamental level, we are led to consider the ways in which the body and brain need to work together to coordinate your health and healing.

Think of your body as a house. All the electricity that comes into the house first has to go through a fuse box, which acts as a distributor of this electricity, sending wires out to different parts of the home to light up the living room, run the refrigerator, and so on.

The chiropractic perspective, its philosophy, is founded on the belief that a vital life force runs through all of us, known as *Innate Intelligence*; and similar to the electrical wiring in your house, it empowers the body to function and to heal.

Your body has nerves running to practically every cell of every organ and tissue, providing vital energy, communication, and healing. That's how the brain controls the rest of the body.

Physical, mental, and chemical stressors can cause interference with this flow, just like when a problem with a fuse creates interference with the flow of electrons through your house wires.

Removing interference with this vital flow through chiropractic adjustments—which can take place in many ways, depending on which one of the many chiropractic techniques is used—is central to the philosophy of chiropractic.

Some chiropractic techniques use a fair amount of force, while others employ a light touch. You need to find the one that works best for you. Some approaches put primary emphasis on the proper function of the joints of the spine and the extremities mainly through biomechanical considerations, including nerves, joints, fascia, muscle, and other connective tissue. Others put more of their attention on the concept of adverse mechanical spinal cord tension patterns, focusing on the fluid neurodynamics of our spinal cord, which is pliable, stretching and bending as we move.[1,2,3,4] Among these are techniques help the body and mind to become more aware of and create internal strategies to dissipate these patterns of tension and dysfunction.

The concept of hidden connections that affect our ability to recuperate from health challenges also applies to the therapeutic approach involved. In chiropractic, experienced clinicians often find areas of silent dysfunction that may not be near where the patient is experiencing discomfort. Finding and addressing those hidden areas can often restore function and ease to painful areas of the body elsewhere. For example, my experience is that chronic neck pain, in particular the type that continues to reappear after different types of therapy, stretching, and massage have been tried, often is a consequence. There are hidden connections to be explored that, when found and acted on, usually bring relief and greater function.

Many of these people suffering from recurring neck pain, with no evidence of disk or nerve dysfunction on MRIs, feel better when I work on other parts of the body—for example, the thoracic area or the first rib. Our musculoskeletal function does not consist of isolated parts. There is a systemic integration within the soft tissues of our bodies that, when dysfunctional, creates symptoms in places that don't seem related.

Even at the level of the soft tissues of our bodies, we experience ourselves as systemic, connected chains of function. Our connective tissue, muscles, and nerves are entwined like a spider's web; tension and tautness in one place has tonal effects throughout the body. It's an application to the body of Buckminster Fuller's tensegrity mode, which is based on the continuity and the integrity of a structure based on its elements of tension.

As a doctor of chiropractic, I pay particular attention to the proper functioning of the nervous system, helping to remove any nerve interference that might affect the body's Innate Intelligence, its self-healing ability.

Doing so helps the brain and body's ability to observe itself, communicate, and self-regulate, so that better health can be achieved and maintained.

The chiropractic philosophy that I'm talking about, which dates back over a century, speaks of a Universal Intelligence. It is a term for what many might call the life force. However you envision it, chiropractic philosophy's main tenet is that this force endows our existence with an intelligent design, and that this force flows through our nerves.

It is akin to what some would call the life force of the universe, sustaining all life. Chiropractic philosophy is based on the belief that the brain absorbs, transforms, and transmits this universal life force in our brain and through the nervous system. That's what we call Innate Intelligence.

Although we cannot live without a brain, spinal cord, or nerves, all of which constitute the nervous system, you don't need to believe in any of the philosophic tenets to get wonderful results from chiropractic care. For many chiropractors, the nervous system is a special place because we believe that it functions as a conduit for the life force that flows throughout our body and helps us to heal.

Commonality behind Diversity

Many healing arts work with a similar concept—that there is some sort of vital force flowing through the body. Some of these arts date back thousands of years. As exotic as they might appear, they all have a number of things in common. Each one of them helps validate and reinforce this vital aspect of us. This is a common ancient belief that transcends culture and time. Basically, it affirms that we are more than our biology.

For example, one of the principles that chiropractic and the ancient healing systems of India have in common is that both believe in a vital life force. In Japan, it is referred to as *ki*. Other countries have other names, such as *gi* in Korea or *mana* in Polynesia. The Indian healing systems work with what they call *chakras*, which is another word for spinning vortices of energy throughout the body. These chakras are located in the same places where there are large clusters of nerve cells, or *ganglia*, which are a focus of chiropractic health.

What we in chiropractic call Innate Intelligence, the Indian healing practices and religions know as *prana*, the life energy. According to their philosophy, prana activates the body and the mind, and manifests in the body as five elements.

The practice of yoga and its associated spiritual concepts from India were introduced in the 1930s to America by a well-known author and teacher named Paramahansa Yogananda. In a chapter titled "Healing Body, Mind, and Soul" from his book *Scientific Healing Affirmations*, Yogananda wrote: "By fasting, massage, osteopathic treatment, chiropractic adjustment of the vertebrae, yoga postures, and so on, we might help to remove or relieve congestion in the nerves or vertebrae and permit the free flow of life energy."[5]

The life energy that I have been referring to in the philosophy of chiropractic has much in common with the energy at the center of other vitalistic healing approaches around the world and through the ages. One reason for this is that throughout many cultures there has existed an almost universal belief that we are spiritual beings expressing physical, emotional, mental, and spiritual dynamics—in other words, the human condition.

In this context, the nervous system is regarded by many as a functional physical bridge between who we are and how we express ourselves physically, emotionally, mentally, and spiritually. It's as if each one of these parts, or dynamics, is represented by one of our fingers, while the nervous system is represented by the palm and the arm that connects to and expresses that central part of us: our essential self.

Chiropractic's main focus is on the body's ability to regain and maintain health aided by this life force, using the spinal cord and the nerves as conduits, along with proper structural function and nerve tone.

Acupuncture is a part of the ancient healing system of China, originating about 2,500 years ago. It was founded on the principle that every living body is endowed with a life force, *chi*, which flows through the body, using channels, or *meridians*, to do so.

Placing needles in some of the more than 2,000 acupuncture points has many beneficial effects on our health. Like chiropractic, acupuncture aims to help remove anything that might be blocking the free flow of this life force throughout the body. Research has shown that one of its main clinical effects, similar to chiropractic adjustments, is to modulate the function of the nervous system.[6]

As you can see, there are core similarities between Eastern and Western healing approaches, although at a more superficial level they might seem unrelated—like different parts of our bodies.

Philosophy, Art, and Science

Often when I am engaged in conversation on this topic, someone asks whether all this can be proved. Many say it just sounds like an unprovable theory—and they have a point. Let's take a closer look at this issue.

Every branch of the healing arts has three legs: philosophy, science, and art.[7]

1. You can think of the first leg—philosophy—as those fundamental beliefs that cannot be proved, such as whether you believe in love, or God, or the power of open minds and hearts.
2. The second leg—the science aspect—is essentially what research is able to demonstrate to be true.
3. The third leg of any healing field—the art—is the skill, the experience, and the techniques that a clinician applies best to that patient.

The philosophy of chiropractic has an interesting history that dates back to the late 1800s. The pioneers of the field believed that this Innate Intelligence, this life force that I mentioned earlier, expresses itself through the spinal cord in the form of what they called "mental impulses."

Emerging science is now pointing in the direction of this connection. Scientists have found that in the spinal cord there is something they call a "mini-brain" that helps to process how we maintain our innate ability to balance.[8]

Another study has demonstrated that the spinal cord processes information similarly to the way parts of our brain do.[9]

Personally, I believe in this chiropractic philosophy—that there's a spirit of life flowing through our nervous system that animates our bodies and its functions. Philosophy, by its nature, cannot be proved. So these are just beliefs, and everyone is entitled to his or her own opinion.

Interesting research is, however, beginning to demonstrate the merit of these chiropractic pioneers' beliefs. Science is always catching up to theory. For example, there is a structure located deep in our brain called the *thalamus*, which works as a relay and processing center, as well as regulating consciousness, among other things. Scientists are discovering more complex levels of just how central it is to brain function.

One such discovery has revealed that the thalamus emits pulsations that travel to all the cells of the body and helps regulate brain waves.[10,11,12,13,14,15,16,17,18,19,20,21] This research is showing that these brain waves affect how brain cells function. Thus, the century-old chiropractic belief that mental impulses originate in the brain and travel through all the nerves in the body now has a scientific parallel.

The person who founded chiropractic said that it was based on tone, and now research is showing that groups of brain cells create patterns of resonance, of tonality, to help communicate with other brain cells. Researchers are noting that biochemical processes alone cannot account for certain long-distance aspects of brain communication.[22]

One of the processes involves brain cells vibrating and entraining other cells at a distance to do so as well.[23] Neurophysiologists named this phenomenon *Mexican waves*, because some brain cells start the process and then others join in, like a wave at a soccer stadium!

The emerging field of neural resonance addresses this and other dynamics. Obviously, more research needs to be done, since science is always playing catch-up with reality...and philosophy.

One of the central aims of this book is to highlight connections between systems and tissues in our bodies that affect the function as well as the state of health of seemingly unrelated parts. Let's take a look at some of the important connections between your spine and health issues that we have research on. We will explore those that go beyond the usual spinal pain or muscle ache.

Before we do that, I'd like to share an observation that comes from my experience working with many thousands of patients throughout the years: When our nervous system, which is composed of our brain, spinal cord, and nerves, is more healthy and in a state of decreased tension, we do more than simply handle the physiological challenges of life better. We also seem to be able to be more aware of the subtle things in our daily lives that come up, and to be able to respond to them in ways that save us from more of life's wear and tear down the road.

You'd be surprised to learn what some of the research has shown regarding the connection between of the function of your spine, which is a part of your nervous system, and illnesses that you might characterize as unrelated.

Much more research needs to be done to bring to light further connections. However, here is a partial synopsis of some of the research involving spinal dysfunction and illnesses: In a study involving 150 unselected cases of developmental heart disorders, according to research published in an osteopathic journal, over 90 percent of the patients had thoracic spinal or paraspinal aberrations in structure and function. Nerves from that area of the spine go to the heart. Cardiac issues often showed up months or years after spinal thoracic dysfunction.[24]

Using brain PET scanning, improved brain function, relaxation, and pain reduction were observed in subjects after chiropractic manipulation of the neck, according to a paper published in a journal of alternative medicine.[25]

An article in a medical journal for ear, nose, and throat specialists revealed that a clinically significant number of patients with hearing disorders caused by spinal dysfunction of the neck, known as *cervicogenic hearing loss*, experienced improved or reversed hearing loss after chiropractic manipulation of the upper part of the neck. Audiometry and otoacoustic emissions were used to measure pre- and postchiropractic treatment changes.[26]

A randomized controlled trial revealed improved crying behavior in infants with colic after chiropractic therapy, according to the *Journal of Manipulative and Physiological Therapeutics*.[27]

A study of 360 patients with allergic disease issues revealed that there may be a strong correlation between thoracic vertebrae deformities and allergic diseases. According to the research, published in a journal of orthopedic surgery, spinal-correction treatment improved skin conditions in over half of the treated patients.[28]

For those who suffer from *irritable bowel syndrome* (IBS), in a study of 210 patients with IBS, half of them received spinal manipulative care, and the other half were given prescription medicine. In a study reported in a journal of traditional Chinese medicine, of the 120 who received the spinal adjustments, 92 reported excellent improvement in their symptoms, and no one reported poor results. Of the other 120 who were on a common drug prescription for IBS, 30 had excellent results, and 22 had poor results. The researchers concluded that the function of the mid- and low-back spine was a contributing factor in irritable bowel syndrome.[29]

Upper abdominal pain is connected to back pain, according to gastroenterologists who examined hospital patients with upper abdominal pain. Patients with upper abdominal pain were four times more likely to complain of back pain. Of those, spinal abnormalities were found on physical examination 75 percent of the time.[30] Of further interest, they found that heartburn was also significantly related to back pain.

Improving the health of our spine through chiropractic adjustments can aid in the recovery from these and other conditions not usually associated with chiropractic care.[31–127]

In looking at just some of these studies, you can see how a function of your body, in this case your spinal health, that at first blush would not seem related to a number of conditions or illnesses, may play a central role in illness and in healing.

It's another instance of this wonderful, interconnected web of life that lies within each of us!

What You Can Do Now

- For many, bigger steps to healing take place when they receive therapies that address the neuromuscular and soft-tissue components of the body. One of them, chiropractic, helps to remove nerve interference so that our body can function more optimally, allowing what many call the body's Innate Intelligence to express better health.
- If the treatment programs you have tried have not been helpful, consider trying a clinical approach that is vitalistic. That is, one that works to release the flow of that inner current, or energy, that we all have. Remember that the body is connected in ways beyond the understanding of science. There may be some approaches that you have not considered that may be clinically helpful.

[8]

The Internet, Blood Pressure, and Emotions

I'VE DISCUSSED HOW our current health care system mirrors an industrially based model—that it treats our bodies largely as machines. And that our bodies are too complex, too dynamic, to be treated as mechanical objects. Our clinical approaches need to reflect and to embrace the interwoven, immediate-response, multicausal structure of our 21st-century world societies and economies.

The Internet has become, in a manner, our global nervous system. Everything is connected, changes are often instantaneous, and many things that occur on the other side of the world can now make an immediate difference for us locally.

Seeing the Internet and other modern communication tools through this perspective gives us technological clues as to how we should be looking differently at our health concerns. This interconnected aspect of the Internet reflects how nature and our bodies function at deeper levels. Just as in a garden, everything is connected and affects each other in some way.

Along those lines, a chiropractic adjustment can do more than just relieve aches and pains. It can help to improve physiology by correcting the structure and function of our bones and our soft tissue, including our nerves. By helping to improve function and remove interference in the spine and nerves of the body, we usually see positive changes, no matter what the practitioner's or patient's belief system might be.

And these changes can be far-reaching, as we will see. Essentially, the more profoundly a therapeutic approach modifies our healing systems, the more effects it can have. There are many other wonderful therapeutic approaches that can help our bodies to heal. You simply need to find the right one for you.

For many chiropractors, however, the primary intent is to help clear the path for the flow of this life force through your body so that it can do what it needs to do—help you to heal.

As I mentioned earlier, health can be analogous to a yellow traffic light—not bad enough to be flashing red, warranting a classical diagnosis and treatment in a health care system that emphasizes crisis or red-flag care. At the same time, it's frustrating to know that your body is telling you that it's not in a green-light status. You know that something's not right—you feel it.

Just because you're not sick in the classic, clinical sense—meaning there is no available evidence of disease—doesn't mean that the 12 systems of your body are working well.

Lack of evidence is not evidence of lack. You might have subclinical issues—in other words, dynamics not picked up by the standard testing parameters. And there might be subtle connections between dysfunctional body systems that could have a cumulative effect and end up causing a lot of discomfort for long periods of time, later leading to the emergence of diseases.

High Blood Pressure

Recently, a patient named Diane spoke to me about her husband. "Doc," she said, "can you tell me how using these health traffic-light colors can have an effect on someone's blood pressure?"

This had been a concern of hers for quite some time. Her husband had not been able to get off his blood pressure medication. In fact, his doctor had increased the dosage again the previous year, and now she wondered about unknown side effects.

She said, "I would love it if Dave could eventually stop taking the medications for his high blood pressure, or at least start reducing them. He's been told to watch his diet and to get off salt. He may not need to do more exercise, because he works very hard physically throughout the day."

I explained to her that drugs are usually administered to make a function of the body go faster or slower. For example, if patients are depressed and have no energy, doctors prescribe something for that set of symptoms, and if patients are anxious, they prescribe something else to get the opposite effect.

"It's a little like the accelerator and the brake in your car," I said. "The vast majority of drugs work either to hit the brake or press on the accelerator to produce a desired effect on the body."

I added that nothing was wrong with taking such drugs. In fact, they should be taken when appropriate. What we are looking at, however, is the bigger picture. We want to place health issues in a larger context, because it will give us a better opportunity to heal if we do so. We are exploring the context in which medicine is used.

In doing so, one important question to ask is what other dynamics are taking place in our body that are impeding normal function and our return to health. I think that it's here where the garden metaphor works so well, where all of our connected tissues and functions have to work well together to produce good health—or a juicy tomato.

This is especially important with high blood pressure, known as *hypertension,* since it is the leading health-related risk of death in the world. One in three adults in the United States has high blood pressure, and another one in three adults has pre-hypertension.[1,2,3] This means that most adults in the United States either have hypertension or pre-hypertension.

Even mildly elevated blood pressure can shorten life expectancy. Hypertension is the most important preventable risk factor for premature death, worldwide.

Blood pressure is a highly variable dynamic in the human body, in that it changes quickly. I've seen many patients' usual blood pressure show a higher reading when they are in my clinic. It's known as "white-coat hypertension." Even if you wait a little and take the blood pressure test again a few minutes later, it might still not give a true indication of what a person's blood pressure pattern is. Many factors can affect such readings.

The American Heart Association recommends that people with high blood pressure monitor it at home so that the patterns of their readings can be followed to better effect. These readings can then be presented to the patient's doctor so that the doctor has more accurate information to better determine how to best help the patient.

In our clinic, we give patients a blood pressure journal so that they can write down their blood pressure readings at various times of the day for a few days. Research shows that home blood pressure monitoring is more effective for predicting stroke risk than the usual reading taken at the doctor's office. The research also shows that more frequent readings provide a more predictive value. Since most people work during the day, morning and evening readings would be effective.[4]

The best time to monitor blood pressure is usually at night. High blood pressure is really an indicator, a marker for vascular dysfunction, and not a disease. If a doctor was concerned about a patient's high blood pressure as a strong risk factor for cardiovascular disease, one of the best approaches would likely be to use a 24-hour ambulatory blood pressure monitor.[5] It is used more commonly in several countries in Europe than is done in the United States.

By taking this approach, doctors can better identify a patient's blood pressure risk relative to cardiovascular disease.[6,7,8,9,10]

Diane asked me if there was a possibility that her husband could get off of the high blood pressure medication down the road, or at least lower his dosage. I talked to her about applying some of these principles that I had brought up, about looking at the body as a garden, when thinking about her husband's high blood pressure issues.

A master gardener, when directed to a problem patch, I told her, would first examine the rest of the garden to see how everything else was doing and to see what could be helping or harming the plants in question.

I noticed that Diane had stopped slouching in her chair when we spoke about how to help her husband, despite the fact that postural and prolonged sitting problems had been one of the things that brought her in to see me. Instead, she was now sitting up straight and listening intently, and speaking with more energy in her voice.

I have a deep appreciation for patients like her, who in the midst of their healing process also want to find out how to help their families. I've observed, time and time again, that when people direct their attention to helping others, however bad they are feeling, they seem to find a little more energy, a spark that comes from deep within.

What You Can Do Now

- Your high blood pressure is connected to the working of your body, mind . . . and life. Explore through the tools in this book what those connections are and how integrating changes in those dynamics may show up as decreased blood pressure numbers!

- Consider creating a blood pressure journal, taking your blood pressure twice a day for a few days, and bringing it to your doctor to show her, instead of just relying on the reading done at the clinic.

- Chapter 32 has natural tools that have been shown helpful to lower blood pressure, as well as stress. These include breathing exercises and mindful heartbeat feedback.

- The website for the American Heart Association is Heart.org. Go to Conditions, then the High Blood Pressure tab. It will direct you to a video that will show you how and when to take your blood pressure readings at home.

[9]

The Pressure's On

LET'S LOOK AT some of the things that most people think create or contribute to high blood pressure, and discover connections that can help if you or someone you care for suffers from it.

Sometimes high blood pressure increases gradually over the years with no apparent cause. This is known as *essential hypertension,* which simply means that science hasn't been able to determine the mechanisms behind this rise.

For many others, consuming excessive amounts of sodium can raise blood pressure. That's why Dave was told by his doctor to cut back on salt, as well as to make sure that he was eating well and exercising.

However, as many as half of those with high blood pressure who eat a lot of salt with their food do not experience decreased blood pressure when they cut back on salt.[1,2]

They are known as having *salt-resistant high blood pressure.* And if they cut back too much, and if their sodium levels drop too low, that can cause other health issues.[3,4]

As with nature, or a garden, everything in the body needs to be in balance. Interestingly enough, sodium from sources other than table salt, such as sodium bicarbonate, commonly known as baking soda, has been known to help lower high blood pressure and also help the function of kidneys that were damaged due to high blood pressure.[5,6,7,8,9,10,11,12,13,14]

Table salt is a combination of chloride and sodium. It's the chloride that forms part of the salt, not the sodium, that seems to be the big issue.[15,16,17,18,19,20,21,22]

Of course, a large number of studies have pointed to increased salt in the diet as a factor contributing to high blood pressure, and for many, decreased salt consumption forms part of a wise clinical approach. The bigger picture here is that salt, or sodium, does not stand in isolation. Every patient benefits from being aware of the context in which any one factor receives most of the clinical attention and how it may affect him or her differently.

Fruits and vegetables can usually help as well, by alkalizing the body, and studies show that vegetarian diets have been associated with lower blood pressure.[23]

Vegetables and fruits usually are good sources of potassium. I mentioned earlier while discussing osteoporosis that the sodium-to-potassium ratio has markedly changed in the American diet. We have stopped consuming more potassium relative to our sodium intake. That may be one reason why fruits and vegetables can help with high blood pressure, since they are good sources of potassium and are usually alkaline.

Potassium, apart from helping the body to lower acid levels, has a direct role in helping to lower blood pressure. Potassium helps the body to absorb *norepinephrine,*[24] a neurotransmitter that decreases blood flow and constricts your vascular smooth muscles. Lower potassium levels increase your blood pressure,[25] and higher levels decrease it.[26]

Those with kidney issues, with other pathologies, or on certain medications should have their potassium levels checked regularly, since these people may have excessive potassium levels.

I suggested to Diane that taking a look at the bigger clinical picture is important to anyone's health. The sodium and high blood pressure issue, just like everything else concerning our bodies, is more complex than a one-prescription, or even a natural supplement, fit-all approach.

Stress and High Blood Pressure

We discussed other factors that can cause high blood pressure, including emotional stress. That can lead to what is known as *neurogenic hypertension,* which means that the high blood pressure is caused by a dysfunction in the brain and nerves. This type of hypertension does not respond well to the usual diuretics and salt-restricted diets because the increase in blood pressure is not due to increased blood volume. Instead, it is due to increased cell receptor activity, which constricts blood vessels and causes the heart to work more strongly.[27]

Apart from stress or some diseases, nicotine, caffeine, and thyroid issues can be a cause of this type of high blood pressure. High blood pressure can also be caused by too much body weight, which forces the heart to work harder. Not doing exercise can also contribute to high blood pressure, because exercise helps to release a compound, nitric oxide, that is involved in helping to relax the muscles in the walls of the arteries.

High blood pressure can result from multiple causes. In an earlier chapter, I mentioned conditions that were associated with brain fog, lack of motivation, and not being able to plan well, concentrate, or reason, among others.

As we already discussed, the front of the brain, along with other parts of the brain, helps regulate how well the back of your brain sends signals to the digestive system. If the front of the brain, the frontal cortex, is not working well, which is usually indicated by these types of symptoms, the back of the brain might not send the proper signals for the digestive system to work properly.

If the front of the brain is not working well, the nerve signals sent by the back of the brain can also lead to high blood pressure. The brain's output of the chronic-stress hormone cortisol also increases blood pressure.

Causes and Help

Many of the causes of high blood pressure are unknown. Recent research has revealed that inflammation, the brain, and nerves play a larger role than previously thought.[28,29,30]

A research study conducted a few years ago and published in the *Journal of Hypertension* demonstrated that a misalignment of the first of the neck bones is associated with increased blood pressure. Chiropractic adjustments to that area significantly decreased blood pressure readings in patients suffering from high blood pressure, and the results were sustained eight weeks later. This study was conducted using 50 patients, yet none of these patients suffered from neck or back pain.[31]

It's another example of dynamics in the body that seem unrelated but have important connections that can change our health.

We also discussed other factors that could affect Diane's husband's blood pressure, apart from salt intake, eating well, and doing exercise. If some organs, such as the adrenals, kidneys, or liver, aren't working as they should, they could also be risk factors for high blood pressure.[32,33,34]

If the kidneys aren't working well, a blood pressure medication could at times increase a person's blood pressure. In this event, doctors could consider running a blood test to check the person's renin levels, which could help determine which type of high blood pressure medication might work best for him.[35,36]

I discussed with Diane other medications Dave might be taking that could also influence his blood pressure, as well as the possibility of congenital blood vessel issues and other factors, such as diabetes, too much alcohol, and cigarette smoking. Genetics, depression, anxiety, and hostility can also have a strong effect on blood pressure. So can over-the-counter pain relievers and cold remedies.[37,38,39]

We have been taught that small to moderate amounts of alcohol are good for the heart. There has been research associating moderate alcohol use with cardiovascular benefits, including what is popularly known as the "French paradox." Despite high consumption of saturated fats, lower coronary disease rates in France are attributed to their wine-drinking habits. On the other hand, there is also new research showing that alcohol might not provide health benefits to the heart or to cardiovascular health.[40] More studies are on their way as well, and they will have their say. One firmly established fact is that alcohol damages the integrity of the blood-brain barrier, a protective mechanism for the brain.

There are certain foods that research shows can help many people with high blood pressure, as well as foods that we would consider healthy but might have a detrimental effect on blood pressure. Most people are told to eat healthier, to eat more fruits and vegetables, and to cut down on fatty foods, along with salt. Research also indicates that people with high blood pressure might benefit by increasing their intake of foods with omega-3 fatty acids, highly absorbable sources of calcium, magnesium, and vitamin D. The ingestion of beets and the amino acid *arginine* is also helpful.[41,42,43,44,45,46,47]

Simply taking supplements in isolation, or not taking into account the context in which any therapeutic approach is applied, whether it be a natural supplement or drugs or even surgery, misses one of the main points of this book: like nature, our body systems interact in a connected fashion. And how we ingest our nutrients reflects that.

As an example, certain amino acids have been shown to decrease high blood pressure for women as effectively as other lifestyle changes—if the sources of these amino acids are plant-based foods, such as broccoli, lentils, spinach, etc. If the same seven amino acids (arginine, cysteine, glutamic acid, glycine, histidine, tyrosine, and leucine) come from animal sources, the effect was more strongly seen in lowered arterial stiffness, and less so in systolic blood pressure.[48] Either of these two changes is beneficial to your cardiovascular system.

Since high blood pressure can originate from emotional causes, relaxation or stress-handling classes, meditation, prayer, therapy, and relaxation exercises have been shown to be of help in dealing with stress.[49]

Doing so can help normalize levels of cortisol, a hormone that is associated with chronic stress. It constricts the arteries and causes blood pressure to increase. It can also lead to stomach ulcers and cause changes in testosterone levels.[50] I suggested to Diane that tests could be run to determine if her husband's cortisol levels were high and contributing to his resistant high blood pressure.

Mind-body approaches that have proved successful in helping to decrease high blood pressure include emotional self-regulation techniques supported by heart rhythm coherence training.[51] These are simple to learn and can be practiced at home.

Stress decreases the birth rate of new neurons in an important part of the brain associated with memory and learning, the hippocampus, while exercise increases the birth rate of these new brain cells, even in older adults.[52]

Beneficial bacteria in fermented foods, such as miso soup, can help with high blood pressure, as can magnesium. Almost half of the U.S. population consumes less than the required amount of this important mineral. Magnesium deficiencies have been associated not only with hypertension but also with type 2 diabetes, osteoporosis, vascular disease, migraines, asthma, and other conditions.[53]

Animal studies have shown that following brain trauma, magnesium levels inside the cells and the blood drop for several days. The bigger the decline in magnesium levels, the worse the prognosis. Traumatic brain axonal injury in animals resulted in a sustained decline in intracellular free magnesium concentration.[54,55]

Another problem associated with magnesium intake levels points to the need for looking at how the body functions interactively, as a work of nature and not in isolation.

People have been taking more calcium supplements than before. Yet most are not aware that the body works best with a balanced ratio of magnesium to calcium. The balance has not been specifically established at a consensus level. During our proverbial caveman days, we ate foods with about the same amount of magnesium as calcium. In the typical American diet, the ratio has been skewed to approximately four parts calcium to one part magnesium.

Increased calcium-to-magnesium intake ratios in the United States over the past 30 years, in food as well as in supplements, have been associated with an increase in type 2 diabetes. Moreover, a deficit in magnesium at a cellular level can create an inflammatory cascade even in the absence of trauma or pathogens.[56,57] Finland, which has one of the highest ratios of calcium to magnesium ingested in the world, also leads the world with the highest incidence of heart attacks in middle-aged men. Having said that, there may be a number of other variables involved. Young adults either taking magnesium supplements or having more magnesium in their diet have a lower likelihood of developing metabolic syndrome.[58]

The addition of magnesium can lower levels of inflammatory proteins such as tumor necrosis factor α and nuclear factor κβ.[59] Tumor necrosis factor inhibitors are prescribed to help with arthridities and immune-related disorders, so magnesium may be of help. So is the spice *curcumin*. Magnesium has also been found to work well for a number of people suffering from migraines.[60]

Lab-Test Limitations

We have discussed the limitations of blood tests before: Blood magnesium levels might be normal, yet less than 2 percent of your magnesium stores are found in extracellular spaces, such as your blood; 98 percent of them are found in the bones and inside your cells. You might show normal magnesium blood levels on your blood tests but not have enough magnesium in your cells for them to function normally.[61] A number of other mineral and vitamin blood tests also have this type of limitation in revealing cellular deficiencies.

Keep this in mind: what is in your blood may not be in your cells. Later we will see how this may be due to a condition millions of women are suffering from, thyroid dysfunction.

Sometimes blood tests simply don't find what's in your body, even if it has been there for years.

A friend of mine had blood samples that came back fine for years. When he underwent valve-repair surgery for his heart, the surgeon found bacterial overgrowth in the back of the valve, saying it had likely been there for quite some time.

I also let Diane know that there was something very simple that Dave could consider doing that has had wonderful results for patients with high blood pressure. It also has been used for thousands of years around the world to provide better health in the broadest sense of the word, spiritually as well as physically.

One of the largest drops in blood pressure ever measured was in a group of 174 people undergoing a clinical trial. It took place without the use of medicine, herbs, or even food.

How did they do it?

All it took was water.

Really . . . just water.

In a clinical trial of clinically supervised water-only fasting, an average drop of 60 systolic points in blood pressure readings was experienced by those with very high blood pressure. All of the subjects were off blood pressure medication by the end of the study. That included a number of people who had started the trial with an average systolic blood pressure reading above 170.[62,63]

This was not a months-long approach. The study involved 11 days of supervised, water-only fasting-off phase. The body can change that quickly if it is given the opportunity. Before you try it, you should consult with your doctor to see if you are a good candidate. More information on this study can be found at healthpromoting.com.

This goes to show the importance of finding connections that can be effective for treating high blood pressure and not just being prescribed pills for a lifetime—which many patients are.

Your Heart Rate: An Important Measure of Your Health

One of the reasons why it is so important to bring down high blood pressure is because it can lead to cardiovascular diseases, including strokes and aneurysms. Remember that in the U.S., two out of three adults have hypertension or prehypertension.[64] Most people who suffer their first stroke or heart attack have high blood pressure.[65,66]

There is another dynamic related to the cardiovascular system that few pay much attention to, yet it's been shown to be a strong indicator for death, whatever the cause.

It's part of a panoramic approach of viewing everything that could be connected to heal a condition or improve a health status, and not just a number or a body part in isolation.

In this case, it has to do with how quickly your heart beats, known as your *heart rate*, or pulse.

Extensive research shows that men with a heart rate higher than around 60 beats a minute have increased rates of dying. The higher the heart rate, the higher the rate of mortality. The same applies for women, except that their heart rate is typically a few beats per minute faster than a man's, so the baseline number is adjusted accordingly.[67,68,69,70]

You may wonder, "Yeah, but what if I work out and have a slim waistline—does it still apply to me?"

It does. In fact, the evidence shows that whether people are in shape or out of shape, are overweight or of normal weight, have cardiovascular disease or any other type of disease or not, increased heart rate is an independent risk factor. And it is not just an association; it's also a causative factor.[71]

"Therefore, attention should be paid not only to your husband's high blood pressure but also to his heart rate," I said to Diane. When we give patients a blood pressure diary, we also ask them to record their heart rate.

Many species in nature also exhibit this phenomenon, of increased heart rates with shorter lifespans.[72,73,74] It's another example of how our bodies function as a reflection of nature. The more we observe nature, the more we can learn about our health.

Anxiety, stress, and physiological challenges such as infections or other conditions can increase our heart rate, which is controlled by our nervous system. One way to help bring down your heart rate naturally is to put attention on breathing more slowly and deeply, from the diaphragm.

When you feel stressed, and have some time during the day (you can do this in the car or at a business meeting—nobody will notice!), practice breathing at fewer than 10 breaths per minute. Focus on bringing your breath farther down than usual toward your belly button while relaxing and expanding your tummy. This will help you to breathe using more of your diaphragm, which will bring more oxygen to your body.

Have you ever noticed the many statues of the smiling Buddha with a rotund belly? It may be more than just fat—he knows the wisdom of breathing from the belly!

The herb *Rhodiola rosea* (there are many other types of rhodiola, but rosea is the type that is used in almost all of the clinical trials) has been found to help to lower the heart rate.[75,76,77] Also consider consuming calcium, omega-3 fatty acids, potassium, and magnesium.

Chiropractic adjustments to the thoracic area of the spine have been shown to lower the pulse rate as well as blood pressure shortly after the adjustments, according to a randomized clinical trial involving 290 patients.[78] Another study demonstrated that neck spinal manipulations significantly lowered heart rates and also significantly improved heart-rate variability readings.[79] Heart-rate variability measures the way in which your heart beats and gives important clinical information about your health.

These and other research results highlight the danger of a tunnel-focused, one-parameter diagnostic clinical approach. If you help everything else in your garden of health to function better, then whatever is there has a better chance of doing well. That includes food, natural supplements, and medications.

This is because your body is more than ready to handle the equivalent of either natural or chemical seeds, and to nurture their effects. It would also more efficiently break down what is no longer needed, such as metabolites, which are the products of chemical transformations in your body—residues of medicines in our system, for example. It's the equivalent of good drainage in a field.

Diane also asked me to touch on the issue of her husband not noticing how she and her son were feeling at times. She said that she thought it was only because of pressure from work and wondered how it could be tied into his high blood pressure.

I explained that research has shown that people with high blood pressure can have more difficulty being aware of the emotional cues of the people around them—even their loved ones. They are more likely to misinterpret or not be aware of what others' expressions are trying to communicate.[80,81,82] The health-garden paradigm includes the mind and emotions, not just physical processes, and includes other aspects as well. But these aspects are related and can affect each other in subtle and complex ways.

She asked, "So, if I understand you right, you are telling me that Dave might not be picking up on our son's quiet distress signals due to his high blood pressure?"

"That's right," I responded. "However, there can be other factors. Remember, everything is connected—one way or another."

What You Can Do Now

- Fruits and vegetables can usually help to lower blood pressure, by alkalizing the body, and studies show that vegetarian diets have been associated with lower blood pressure. Potassium, apart from helping the body to lower acid levels, has a direct role in helping to lower blood pressure.

- If a prescription for high blood pressure is indicated, a renin blood test may be helpful in determining which type of blood pressure medication may work best for you.

- High blood pressure induced by stress does not respond as well to diuretics and food changes. Consider sessions with an appropriate type of therapist for further help.

- Research indicates that people with high blood pressure might benefit by increasing their intake of foods with omega-3 fatty acids, highly absorbable sources of calcium, magnesium, vitamin D, beets, and the amino acid arginine. Beneficial bacteria in fermented foods, such as miso and sauerkraut, can help with high blood pressure, as can magnesium.

- Fasting has been clinically proved to have a significant and quick effect on high blood pressure. Visit healthpromoting.com for more information.

[10]

Everything Is Connected, Everything Matters

DIANE AND I spent some time talking about the mind-body connection.

I explained to her that by doing everything possible to assist his body's natural healing ability to regulate itself, her husband had a better chance of having a body that worked the way it was supposed to. When that happened, his blood pressure levels would have a much better chance to normalize, which could in turn help him to be more attentive to the emotional needs of his family.

I mentioned that the field of biopsychosocial medicine is relatively new. Science now knows that neurotransmitters and chemical messengers associated with emotions are found not just in the brain but also throughout the body.[1]

The principles of a mind-body connection, however—of a unified whole—go back to antiquity. And well they should, because this connection reflects how nature works. Society has shifted again quite a bit in the last few decades. The practice of medicine in the past century was largely mechanically driven, microscopically focused, and molecularly inspired. But our culture, the way we interact with others, is leaving that traditional mechanistic paradigm behind. The present is about wide-ranging connections, immediacy, communication, complexity, and the growing awareness of how the distant affects the local.

It's not a coincidence that this is how nature and our bodies work. Our steps forward in technology and communication are also a reaffirmation and reconnection with the dynamics of nature and of health. If our clinical approaches start to catch up with the way our society now functions, we will be taking big steps forward in understanding how our bodies work and how to better help ourselves to heal.

Clinically, we are beginning—being forced, actually—to look beyond antibiotics as a virtual cure-all. As we enter the post-antibiotic era of health care, medical care is being pressed, out of necessity, to take a page from our past and look into taking a closer view of the functions of the systems within our bodies in relation to each other, to our environment, and to our food. Basically, the call is to look with an integrated perspective at what has been approached largely mechanically and segmentally.

That shift may take many years to come to fruition. Meanwhile, a big-picture perspective can help you make better choices for you and your family in the years to come, with or without the advice of a health professional. It can guide you to better health choices.

First, let's recap some of the main points we have touched on so far.

- The increase in prescription drug use for young and old was discussed.
- The concept of a garden was introduced as a metaphor for how the body works.
- Symptoms as consequences of the body's experiencing barriers to healing were reviewed.
- We talked about the connection between digestion and depression.
- Our health care model is based on a viewpoint that largely treats the human body as a machine, mirroring the paradigm of the Industrial Revolution. We covered how we have moved away from a more natural, all-encompassing approach to health.
- The 12 systems of the body were highlighted.
- A traffic light was suggested as a metaphor for our general health status: green, yellow, or red.
- We explored chiropractic and other vitalistic philosophies, and what they had in common: the individual beyond biology and the principle of an energy or life force running through each one of us, as described throughout the ages in various ways by different cultures in their healing approaches.

In looking for the big clinical picture, the one that will yield the biggest impact on our health, I have found, interestingly enough, that the biggest challenge is usually in asking the right types of questions.

Here is a story that illustrates that.

I briefly studied with a doctor who had traveled from the United States to a remote village in India to work with another doctor. This doctor was widely known for being knowledgeable in an ancient diagnostic and healing discipline—pulse reading. When the young doctor arrived at the remote village after his long journey, he was told to rise early in the morning and walk along a narrow, winding path through the forest. There, in a small group of huts, he would meet his new teacher.

He got up early the next morning and was offered a breakfast consisting of *paratha*—a type of unleavened flatbread stuffed with vegetables—and some tea. He was eager to start and quickly made it to his teacher's modest dwelling.

Upon arriving, he was graciously greeted by his new mentor, who offered him tea and asked him to sit down. After some polite conversation, the doctor asked the traveler if he had any questions. The young man responded that he hadn't thought of anything to ask, saying that he was simply there to learn at the feet of his teacher.

The wise mentor smiled ruefully at the eager doctor, who had traveled many thousands of miles to be with him, and gently told him to go away, and not to return, unless he first thought of what questions to ask.

The young doctor, confused and disappointed, got to his feet and slowly trudged on the long, dusty walk back to the village, with much to think about.

While he was walking on the brown clay road, he reflected on the wisdom of this approach and returned early the following morning, ready with questions. During the length of his training with this teacher, he later told me, he received instructions only after asking a question.

What I learned from this doctor's story was that asking the right questions can be more important than the answers themselves. If you aren't ready to ask the question, the answer will be of lesser use, or perhaps of no use at all. The young doctor's teacher knew this and wanted to make sure that he taught his student what he was ready to grasp and to apply.

True Doctoring

In a literal sense, this teacher was doctoring. Most people are not aware of the derivation of the word *doctor*. It comes from the Latin for "teacher." Ironically, the knowledge that comes from teaching is many times the biggest help to healing, rather than drugs or surgical procedures.

People look for things to help them feel better, but in doing so they can miss out on the fundamentals of health and healing. An increasing number of people are realizing that we will benefit more from applying nature and life principles in caring for our health.

It takes time for a society to change. Meanwhile, through the use of this book, you can move to the front ahead of the usual learning and growth curve and more easily experience better health.

Health care models follow economic models, although in a quickly changing society there is usually a lag time until both are on the same proverbial page. I believe that's what is happening to us now. While we wait and encourage the rest to catch up, let's do what we can to benefit from this shift individually. We'll discuss more about how you can do that shortly.

Emerging technologies have made us more aware that our planet and our connected economies depend on and affect each other, even when geographically remote. Another paradox is that modern science, in learning more about the atomic and subatomic realms, is enabling us to be more aware of the closely knit relationships between all things on our planet, including the small and the distant. This parallels ancient cultural and tribal wisdoms about how our bodies work.

We are much more aware, for example, of how environmental conditions in one distant part of the planet can affect us here at home. However, this isn't news to our bodies, because our bodies have always worked this way, whether we have been aware of it or not.

One example of this is your brain.

What You Can Do Now

- One of the most important first steps in helping yourself and your loved ones is to formulate the right questions.

- That determines how you will approach an issue. For example, instead of asking yourself, what do I take for this, even if it is organic or "natural," consider asking yourself, what has happened that has placed my body in a situation where I need it to begin with? What processes or functions are not working as they should, and what could be the causes? What can I do to support my body to correct those underlying barriers or deficiencies? Whom can I ask to help me with that, or where can I find answers?

- The way you frame your questions frames how you approach your issues. Look for secondary as well as primary causes of issues.

[11]

It Takes a Village

OUR BRAIN IS multimodal, meaning that the brain cells, or neurons, work as a community and depend on the communication of other groups of brain cells to keep them functioning well. Every part of the brain needs to interact with other parts of the brain in order to develop normally and for all of its parts to function well.[1,2,3]

For every one of the neurons in our brain, there may be as many as 10 supporting cells that help with its function. In effect, it takes a neural village.

Our brain also needs communication, coordination, and a sense of functional community from other parts of the body in order to work well. Systems in your body help each other to work better, just like the brain.

Jennifer was a middle-aged patient whose problems included memory issues and difficulty concentrating. She thought her brain was just tired and not working well because she was getting older.

I suggested that age was not the reason and that the problems with her brain function could have started outside her brain.

How Your Thyroid and Brain Affect Each Other

We discussed the connections between her brain and her thyroid. She knew that her thyroid gland could affect her weight and energy levels but was not aware of the extent to which it could affect brain function—and vice versa.

Here is part of what I shared with her: Your thyroid is a gland in your neck that takes its name from the Greek for "shield," because of its shape. Your thyroid releases hormones throughout the body that affect many other functions, including regulating body temperature, metabolism, and brain development during childhood. It helps to control how sensitive your body is to other hormones, as well as a number of other important things. We'll cover some of those in a minute; for now, let's start with hormones.

What are hormones? Think of them as molecular compounds that work as messengers—like telegrams. They are biochemical-signaling molecules that inform cells about what needs to be done. They do so by attaching to cell receptors.

In terms of how they work, picture a series of locks on your front door. Each lock represents a specific cell hormone receptor. The particular biochemical structure of the hormone is like a key that fits that particular lock, or receptor. It's more complex than that, but for purposes of illustration, it will do.

Receptors for thyroid hormones help start a chain of processes within the cell to produce the right type of cellular response, such as manufacturing needed proteins. And since there are thyroid receptors in your brain cells, thyroid dysfunction can affect memory and brain function when your thyroid brain receptors are not stimulated properly.[4,5,6]

Most people think that the brain controls everything. In reality, the body, including the brain, works like our garden metaphor. Different aspects affect each other in intricate ways that we have not fully discovered. Thyroid problems can affect the brain, including causing memory and attention problems like Jennifer's.

However, as in all deeply interconnected open systems it's not always that simple! We're working with the complexity of nature. You can have the symptoms of, say, an underactive thyroid, yet the lab-test screening for thyroid hormones can come back normal. I see this often in my clinic during screening tests. It happened with Jennifer, who was frustrated with not knowing what to do when her blood workup came back negative but she continued not feeling well.

I asked Jennifer how many other times she, her family, or her friends went to see a doctor because they had a number of things that were affecting them, but when blood tests were run, all that was found was a slightly high level of cholesterol or slightly elevated blood sugar.

She replied that this was one of the things her mother complained about. Her mother was frequently tired and achy, didn't have much energy, had digestion problems like Jennifer, and often did not sleep well. But the lab tests always came back normal, and the doctors would tell her that nothing was showing up as "wrong." So they prescribed a painkiller or an antacid for her stomachaches, or something to help her sleep.

Keep this in mind the next time your doctor looks at your blood test results and says you're fine: Your blood weighs around 13 pounds, less than 10 percent of your weight. How's the other 90 percent functioning?

Additionally, lab tests usually test for a disease or a well-defined illness. Many doctors are highly trained to work with pathology, but are usually not well-trained or educated to work with subtler issues, such as subclinical organ dysfunctions that might need attention through natural approaches rather than with prescription medicine.

The challenge is that unfortunately, not much research has been done in this field. Research is expensive, and the majority of published studies focus on pharmacological approaches. For many chronic health issues, by the time something shows up on a lab test as abnormal, the patient has been losing his health for some time. He's usually been complaining that something has been wrong with him for a while.

The tests that many patients undergo are designed to find problems with structure or pathology; but to the detriment of the patients, they are not usually designed to pick up subtler clues of dysfunction.

Jennifer asked me if I could provide her with examples.

I shared with her what happens often with a number of imaging studies, and took MRI as an example. Typical MRI results might not tell the whole story, although they provide doctors with high-resolution images of the body. Many times, patients with strong lower back pain receive MRI results that show no pathology of note. Those MRIs are usually done with the patient lying down, which is how they are performed most of the time.

When weight-bearing MRI exams are done, with the patient standing, disk pathology that was not seen in the usual reclining MRI results often shows up. People suffering from low back pain while standing who have had MRIs performed while lying down and have been told that nothing abnormal was found may want to consider asking their treating physician about upright, or orthostatic, MRI testing. A radiological study involving more than 4,300 people over a 10-year period revealed a significant number of occult low back spine and disc pathologies that were not present in recumbent MRI findings.

MRI changes in the upright position that were not present when patients were lying down were found 68 percent of the time.[7] Meniscal tears of the knee have also been discovered more often in weight-bearing MRIs than in recumbent ones.[8]

We discussed another example that was closer to home, thyroid blood test results. Patients often have a blood test that shows normal reference levels of a common hormone used to measure thyroid function—the thyroid-stimulating hormone (TSH). However, research has shown that high-normal levels in both men and women are associated with weight gain.[9,10]

TSH levels can appear normal on lab tests, yet in the presence of a pituitary tumor some of this hormone might be biologically inactive, decreasing thyroid function, while showing normal on the blood test.

Some of the symptoms of pituitary tumors include visual issues, headaches, tiredness, weight changes, and changes in menstrual cycles. Inflammatory diseases of the intestines, such as celiac disease, or adrenal insufficiency can also affect how well the thyroid works.

It's all part of our intricately connected web of health.

Next, I will tell you how you can help yourself by learning about this little powerhouse of a gland that weights as little as five quarters but that affects almost every function of your body—including your weight!

What You Can Do Now

- If you have continuing challenges with brain function, make sure that your thyroid, and the cells in your body that respond to thyroid hormones, are working as they should.

- Normal blood lab results do not necessarily mean that your body is responding well to your thyroid hormones or other body functions. Remember that your blood weighs only around 13 pounds. There's a lot more of you than that. A blood test is not a full health test.

- Often, a full complement of thyroid testing is not performed. Ask your doctor to look into ordering more thyroid-related testing in case issues are present that are not found with the usual TSH test. We'll discuss this in more detail in the next chapter.

- If you continue to experience symptoms associated with thyroid issues in the absence of red flags on your thyroid lab tests, consult with a specialist to see if your body is not responding well to your thyroid hormone production.

[12]

That Little Gland Does What?

THE THYROID GLAND is situated in the middle of your neck and forms a glandular bridge between your head and the rest of your body.

You might recall that I said that thyroid issues can affect brain function and that you could get lab test results that did not show thyroid issues, but there still could be problems and symptoms associated with your thyroid—such as weight gain.

Dysfunction of the thyroid can also lead to bad digestion, hair loss, tiredness, weak nails, constipation, memory loss, depression, and a number of other symptoms. If you have a thyroid that is working weakly, that alone can increase cortisol levels, which in turn can increase estrogen as well as promote weight gain and inflammation.[1]

Abnormal thyroid hormone levels can also affect calcium absorption, which can increase levels of osteoporosis and lead to a higher incidence of bone fractures. They can also reduce the level of growth hormones necessary for your body.[2]

Your thyroid helps control the rate of metabolism, or the amount of energy used, in your body, which is important for weight loss. Low thyroid hormone levels, even levels considered normal, can often lead to increased weight, diabetes, and high blood pressure.[3]

On the subject of osteoporosis and diabetes, type 2 diabetics have to be careful with this issue. Their bone density tests might show normal or high density levels, but due to the negative impact of this disease on the quality of the microarchitecture of the bone marrow, they are more prone to fractures.[4]

Body Connections

These far-ranging effects are why I chose the thyroid as an example. It goes to the heart of what I have been talking about: this interconnectedness, this whole body-health relationship.

There's a gland in your brain, the hypothalamus, that sends messages to another gland in your brain, the pituitary, which signals the thyroid to produce hormones. This pituitary gland hormone, the thyroid-stimulating hormone introduced in the last chapter, can show up as being at a normal level on a blood test. But it's how your body responds to thyroid hormones, even if lab tests are normal, that is more important.

Every person is unique; no one else has had your life experiences or a body identical to yours. Your health experiences, including how you respond to medications and your internal hormone levels, are unique to you.

How your body reacts can make a significant difference compared with how someone else reacts, even if you have the same thyroid lab-test levels. Most people who have thyroid issues have an underactive thyroid, which is known as a *hypothyroid* condition.

The body depends on the liver and small intestine to activate most of these thyroid hormones so that the body can use them at the cellular level. Therefore, liver or intestinal issues can compromise how your body responds to and uses the hormones made by your thyroid. That is why you can have a normal level of thyroid stimulating hormones on your lab test results, but if your body is not working with them properly, you can still end up with symptoms of thyroid dysfunction.

Patients who are suffering from the symptoms of an underactive thyroid are usually diagnosed as having thyroid dysfunction based on results from lab tests for one or two hormones: thyroid-stimulating hormone, known as TSH, or *thyroxine,* known as T4.

Yet many who are told that nothing is wrong continue to suffer from thyroid-hormone-related problems, such as cold extremities, weight gain, dry skin, menstruation issues, muscle aches, depression, low libido, water retention, and fatigue. Many patients have been prescribed medication such as levothyroxine, a synthetic form of T4, on the basis of these blood tests.

For over 10 years, however, research has been pointing in a more complex direction, one that takes into account a central theme of this book: that what is taking place in other parts of the body affects the symptoms and health of seemingly unrelated functions.[5]

The pituitary gland has a feedback system, like a thermostat, that tells the thyroid when to make more or less of certain hormones, mostly T4. It produces TSH to do so.

However, relying on TSH levels to determine the levels of thyroid hormones in the cells of your body may not be accurate. And that may lead to a wrong diagnosis or incorrect dosage. One of the reasons for this is that the pituitary's feedback system does not always reflect the true levels of active thyroid hormones inside the rest of the cells of your body.[6,7,8]

It's important to note that the thyroid hormone receptors in your pituitary are different from those in the rest of your body.[9] Additionally, the transport system carrying thyroid hormone into your pituitary works differently than it does in the rest of your body. When the rest of your body is under different types of stresses, fewer thyroid hormones make their way into the cells, while the transport system for the pituitary often does not change much.

Therefore, the amount of TSH produced by your pituitary to balance thyroid production may not be a true reflection of what your body's thyroid hormone levels really are. Think of it as being like a faulty thermostat that turns the heat in your home off and on. It works, more or less, but it may not be quite tuned in to your temperature needs.

Yet TSH levels, for many practitioners, remain the cornerstone in determining whether and how much hormone prescription medication to give. Often that is not enough.[10]

Some of the conditions that can drive fewer thyroid hormones into the cells of your body yet show normal blood pituitary thyroid hormone levels include diabetes, high cholesterol, toxins, chronic fatigue, anxiety, and chronic dieting.[11]

The complexity associated with problems involving thyroid hormone, however, go beyond pituitary feedback function. Different types of tissues in your body may have different active hormone levels.

Prescriptions that use only synthetic T4 may not be fully helping those with hypothyroid symptoms if the transport mechanisms for T4 are compromised, which can occur in a number of the conditions mentioned above.

If you suffer from hypothyroid symptoms despite being told that you have normal TSH results, or while taking T4 supplements, talk to your prescribing physician about considering lab testing for free T3/reverse T3 ratios to see what they may tell you about indications of thyroid intracellular problems.[12,13,14,15]

One important takeaway from this topic reminds me of the old saying used in real estate when addressing the issue of land value: location, location, location. The same applies for your thyroid dynamics. Normal levels of tested hormones in the blood are fine, but most important are their levels inside the cells of your body, since this is where your body really responds to their presence.

Also consider inexpensive blood testing for autoimmune issues associated with hypothyroidism, such as Hashimoto's disease, which is the main cause of hypothyroidism in America. While there is no cure for Hashimoto's, there are natural approaches that may help the body to manage autoimmune responses, such as maintaining good levels of vitamin D.

Returning to the discussion of the complexity of the connections in our bodies, excess levels of estrogen, for example, can affect how thyroid hormones work.[16] Excess estrogen can also lead to wanting to eat sugary foods.

Remember that I mentioned the importance of hormone receptors? Active thyroid hormones stimulate receptors in the nucleus of our cells. So these receptors also have to be active and working well. No blood lab tests are commonly used to test for how well these intracellular receptors are working.

The cells that receive your thyroid hormones—and remember that hormones are chemical messengers that tell the cell to take action—have to be healthy. They need to respond appropriately once the nuclear receptors have been activated. If your cells are not working well, even if these thyroid receptors are working normally, they might not respond the way they should.

That's why cellular health is an important factor in overall health. Blood hormone levels might appear normal, but if there is a problem with how the cells respond to hormones, which act as chemical messengers, it's as if someone is trying to deliver a package to your door but no one is home to accept it and benefit from its contents.

That's why people can have normal hormone test results yet have symptoms associated with hormone insufficiency.

Stress Hormone Effects

When you are under chronic stress, your body produces cortisol, the stress hormone that we spoke about earlier. Cortisol can reduce the amount of hormones that your thyroid makes[17] and can also contribute to blocking of progesterone receptors.

Additionally, high cortisol levels make it harder for your body to accept these thyroid hormones, so you can end up having thyroid symptoms even though lab tests show normal hormone levels. Inflammation is another issue that can decrease thyroid function.

Other factors that can cause your thyroid to not function well include environmental toxins, kidney dysfunction, certain types of prescription drugs such as lithium, pregnancy, and a family history of thyroid dysfunction.

It's important to take into account that nutritional deficiencies can be a factor for some people. For others, certain foods, such as products containing gluten, can have an effect on thyroid function.

To help a gland or system to work better, as we have seen, a number of processes and systems have to work together. Here we have highlighted the function of the thyroid gland, which supports brain function and, in turn, is affected by brain function, as well as by a number of other functions in the body. And that's only one of the many glands, organs, and tissues in your body that can have this type of cause and effect.

It might not be enough to simply give a patient thyroid medicine when she has a low thyroid hormone count. The prescribing doctor serves the patient best by looking at the whole body and seeing what connections could be contributing to the problem or can help it to heal.

Are there underlying barriers that are slowing down the body's ability to produce and use that hormone the way it should?

Approximately 45 million people, mostly women, have issues with hypothyroidism. Many don't know even about it.[18] You can have more than one dysfunctional gland, or system, that contributes to a symptom, just as a number of things can be wrong in a garden.

In the end, health is about the body working in an integrated fashion, like nature, or even like members of a community working toward important projects. In some remote villages in primitive societies, for example, everyone in the village, especially the elderly, helps to rear the children. The same applies for the functions of cells and systems in our bodies.

It takes a village at a cellular level as well.

Socrates warned against treating only one part of the body, saying that unless the whole was well, the part could never be well.

More women than men have a sluggish thyroid gland because females produce more female hormones, such as estrogen, that can make it harder for the thyroid to produce the same level of thyroid hormones found in men.

During ovulation, women exhibit a temporary increase in thyroid output, which increases metabolism. You've heard of women taking their temperature to help determine when they are ovulating. Well, during ovulation, there's a spike in body temperature that's associated with a temporary increase in thyroid output, which increases metabolism.[19,20]

Next, we will talk about something that many people do every day, usually at breakfast, thinking it's always a healthy way to start the morning—juicing.

Or is it?

What You Can Do Now

- Bone density tests for type 2 diabetics may not reveal any issues, yet there may be cause for concern. If in doubt, or if a test came back showing issues, consider additional testing with your physician.

- Stress affects how well your hormones can work, including your thyroid and progesterone receptors. If symptoms associated with these show up and you have been under long-term stress, consider stress as a root cause, and address it as well.

- For some, gluten can lead to thyroid-associated symptoms. Getting off gluten for a few weeks and seeing if the symptoms clear up can be one way of establishing whether it is an issue for you.

- Keep in mind that blood testing is not an absolute determinant of whether your body has thyroid issues. Don't assume that because the test came back normal, it means your body has normal thyroid hormone function.

[13]

Problems with Smoothies?

SMOOTHIES AND JUICING are wonderful, yet at the same time, they may not be as good for you as you might think.

Many people love them and drink up to 16 ounces or more every morning. The thought is that if one green vegetable or fruit is good for them, why not a ton of them? And in our bigger-is-better, fast-paced society, why not just drink them instead of taking the time to eat them?

For most people, the best way of eating something is to have it in the form in which nature provided it to us. There's a reason why nature's garden does not provide liquid vegetables!

When we liquefy fruits and vegetables, we usually aren't chewing them. However, digestion should start in the mouth rather than in the stomach. Chewing stimulates nerve centers in the brain that prepare the digestive system, and the saliva produced helps the stomach to digest food better (see chapter 27 for more on the benefits of chewing well).

Chew your smoothies!

When you use a blender or a juicer, you are grinding up a type of fiber, insoluble fiber, which is necessary for good digestion and health. The soluble fiber remains if you use a blender, but the insoluble fiber is pulverized. Insoluble fiber is important, as it can help with constipation and hemorrhoids. Too much soluble fiber can slow the transit time for food in the intestines.

Moreover, insoluble fiber helps you to absorb fewer calories, because the food is delivered deeper in the intestines, where bacteria can absorb some of the calories.

Don't get me wrong—I am not minimizing the great positives for juicing. Despite some issues, juicing has a lot of benefits and could be the best choice for many people, especially those with sensitive digestion or certain digestive diseases. There is research showing good changes in a large number of health issues that are associated with juicing.

But we can lose a number of benefits, depending on when we blend or how we drink the liquid. And if we are not careful, we can put juicing to work against our better health.

Because few of us take the time to chew, we can easily end up drinking a lot of calories with the vegetable and fruit blends. That leads to gaining weight easily if the juices have a lot of sweet fruits to give them a better taste. There is no way that people could eat all the fruits and vegetables that they can swallow in less than a minute when using a juicer or blender.

By simply blending or juicing fruits and some veggies, we are usually not getting much in the way of proteins. Most people are loading themselves with carbohydrates. For most people, I recommend eating protein in the morning, or at least adding a protein powder to your juice. It helps stabilize sugar levels for a lot of people. The soluble fiber in the smoothie also helps with that.

Make sure that you have good fats as part of your breakfast, too. You can put a spoonful of organic coconut oil in the blender, or put half an avocado in, since it is a good source of healthy fats. Approximately 75 percent of the avocado's calories come from fat, most of it monounsaturated. Eating avocados was shown to reduce total cholesterol, increase good cholesterol, and reduce bad cholesterol as well as a form of fat known as *triglycerides*.[1,2]

In any case, it's good to drink the juice or smoothie shortly after making it because the blades break open the cell walls containing the nutrients, and some of the food enzymes break down quickly. Once it's ready, you should chew each mouthful at least a few times before swallowing.

What You Can Do Now

- Chew anything that is not water. That includes smoothies and juices.
- The more you chew your food, the better the digestion, and the less you end up eating.
- Make sure that during the day you also have sources of food that have insoluble fiber, which juicing usually destroys. Insoluble fiber helps with constipation, hemorrhoids, weight loss, and is healthy for your gut.

[14]

Are Your Symptoms Really Consequences?

AS WE'VE SEEN in the examples in this book so far, symptoms are the expression of the body's attempts to heal itself. Acute inflammation is your body's healthy response to a trauma or injury. But if it cannot heal itself, the symptoms become chronic because the body has not completed its full healing cycle. This can lead to conditions such as chronic inflammation, which is a leading cause of diseases.

When you treat a person instead of a symptom, you have a much better chance of helping the body to function better, so that it can self-regulate and heal itself. Our body's fabric is a complex, interwoven pattern. It is, literally, the cellular tapestry of life.

When talking to some patients about certain dietary restrictions, I often notice a strong reluctance to stop eating bread and similar types of foods. This resistance is a consequence of certain eating patterns. There is a reason why so many people respond so forcefully at the thought of eliminating certain foods.

Let's explore some of those connections; it will help you to better understand how to work with your body to lose weight, and to make it easier to eat healthier.

Food is more than just nutrition. A lot more! It affects how our brain works. Take bread, for instance. There are protein derivatives in it that attach to morphine-like receptors in your brain, which alter how your brain works and how you feel. Foods affect moods.

Ever wonder why junk food tastes so good? The texture of food—the combination of fats, salts, sugars, and carbs—is thoroughly studied in expensive laboratories of many fast-food companies to produce the snacks that you find so hard to resist.

Food, in its many varieties, modulates how we feel. It is a big part of the reason why it is so hard for many people to lose weight and to eat well. Why we eat goes far beyond appetite suppression and nutrition.

Your desire for food goes way beyond getting nutrients and feeding your belly. Understanding and addressing this will go a long way to creating easier steps to a better diet.

Digestion and Health

Poor food digestion can have more effects on your health than just indigestion. Let's start with a run-of-the-mill upset stomach as an example; it highlights the importance of understanding how the functions in your body are connected.

Having a tummy ache can affect how your brain works, believe it or not, such as forgetting where you put your car keys or forgetting to buy those other two things when you leave the supermarket. But what's the connection?

We have about 25 feet of intestines in our bodies. The surface area of your small intestine alone is about the size of a tennis court. It's a lot of real estate to keep healthy. When the intestines are stressed, which can be caused by a number of problems, the walls can become more permeable and allow harmful substances to enter the intestines and bloodstream.

Eventually, these harmful substances can end up in the brain and can include bacteria and food particles that cause allergic reactions.[1,2] What happens is that these substances—proteins, pathogens, and inflammatory chemicals—can enter the blood circulation of your brain. Sometimes they are able to go through what is known as the *blood-brain barrier*.

The blood-brain barrier is a protective layer of blood vessels around the brain that helps protect it from foreign particles, like a moat around a castle.

Inflammation in your intestines is associated with a greater chance of inflammation in this protective blood-brain barrier. This can lead to substances entering your brain that aren't good for it. These substances can cause brain inflammation and depression, which we talked about, as well as a decrease in your ability to concentrate. They can also increase the possibility of autoimmune disorders, diabetes, and celiac disease.

Inflammation can affect how your brain works, and so can your thyroid glands, as we have discussed, as well as your adrenal glands. Your digestive, circulation, and immune systems can also affect your brain function. As you can see, many parts of your body are involved in the proper functioning of your brain.

Your body is one big interacting, fluid matrix. High blood pressure can also make this blood-brain barrier more open to toxic substances and infectious agents that may end up in the brain.[3] Additionally, high blood pressure can lead to an increased risk for food allergies as well as diabetes.

It helps to think of your body as a circulating series of connected waterfalls, each influencing the other. A flow of biochemical substances interact with each other and carry information that extends far beyond our body's blood circulatory system. Every system, organ, tissue, and cell in your body touches and interacts with every other part of your body in ways that science has yet to discover, but that still affect our health.

Our bodies have always been doing what society is now recognizing as vital to our economy and lifestyle—communicating and maintaining a relationship with other distant societies in order to maintain a healthy global economy.

In line with this connection, an interesting study showed that there is a similarity in how cities grow—how highways and exits are created as cities expand—and how our brain grows when we are young.[4] The researchers discovered that the appearance of highways and exit ramps in a growing city closely resembles the pattern of nerve connections in a child's developing brain.

This is another example of the patterns of nature being expressed in society. It also applies to how our body functions. The paradox is that the more we progress into the future, the more the future reveals dynamics that look like those in the past, which is how nature has always done things!

Let's take the latest that science has to offer and merge it with traditional concepts from the wisdom of nature-based ancient societies, where everything was seen as interrelated and affecting each other, including our health.

To illustrate this, we will begin with a seed.

What You Can Do Now

- Always remember that food can powerfully modulate your brain function. Before succumbing to the temptation, ask yourself, am I eating that to satisfy my nutrition—or my mood?

- Take a pause, just a few seconds, to ask yourself that. Then ask yourself what else you could eat that would still make you feel pretty good but would be at least a little healthier. This simple approach will go a long way, over time, toward reducing your waist size.

- Little habits, done for a long time, yield BIG results!

- A good way to naturally help your intestines to heal is by taking L-glutamine supplements, or by eating whey protein, for those who can handle it. The same proteins that help to keep the intestinal walls intact are also found in the brain's protective barrier system, so helping the health of one helps the other.

[15]

Seeds of Health

BY VIEWING YOUR body as an interconnected garden, you are resonating with ancient, traditional ways of healing and will have taken an important step toward better health.

If you have a fertile plant seed, whether it is organic or genetically engineered, what are the chances of it taking root if it lands on a rocky, dry surface?

Let's play with this seed metaphor a little more. Have you noticed that most of the medication pills that you have taken, in fact, most of your nutritional supplements for that matter—look a lot like seeds? Think about it: they are small, round, and planted the same way a seed is planted in the ground—by introducing it through an opening, your mouth.

Think of all the prescription pills that you have taken, as well as organic nutritional supplements, as seeds. Picture your body as either moist, fertile soil or the equivalent of a rocky, dry surface. This has been the condition of your body—your internal soil, so to speak—that has determined how you responded to whatever you have taken to help yourself heal.

With a garden, once you plant your seeds, you must patiently wait, making sure that the soil and other conditions are ideal. These seeds then either sprout or don't; this is just like waiting to see if the medicine will work or not. The same goes for supplements, or food, or anything else we enter into our digestive system. We plant the seed inside of us, similar to seeds or bulbs, and then we wait to see if it, in a manner of speaking, germinates. Then, if we can harvest its results, we will experience a robust crop—better health!

Whether we're taking prescription pills, supplements, or even food—whatever we take to try to heal ourselves—we have a better chance of it serving our health needs when our soil—our body—is functioning at its fertile best. Our body is a dynamic, organically based organism that, when healthy, can absorb and interact with what we place in it to give us a better chance of abundant harvests of good health.

This brings up a point; it's where a lot of people get tripped up. They think this applies only to food or natural supplements. However, if a person's condition has progressed to the point where he needs pharmaceutical intervention, then this model works by helping him to prepare his body so that even a strong chemical seed, whether it's prescription medicine, an emergency intravenous source, or even surgery, has a better chance of working the way it was intended, and to recuperate better.

Everything in our body, as in nature or a garden, is connected to each other in some way and creates effects.

Your stomach also acts as a sentry, a gatekeeper, as well as one of the organs for digestion. It helps to kill bugs, such as viruses and bacteria, before they enter other parts of your body. I have already detailed how stomach dysfunction can affect your digestion and your intestines. A healthy stomach helps prepare the liver and pancreas for digestion.

Let's quickly review some of the latest topics that we've touched on:

- Improperly digested food and bugs can cause a strain on your small and large intestines, which can lead to intestinal inflammation.
- Improperly digested food can also lead to permeability of your intestinal walls, so that larger proteins and bugs get into your bloodstream and affect other parts of your body. The parts, unfortunately, include your brain, which can lead to brain inflammation.
- Brain inflammation, in turn, can cause parts of your brain to not work as well, which means these parts have more difficulty regulating other parts of your brain, including the health of your intestines. Brain inflammation can also lead to difficulty concentrating, moods, and memory issues.

A vicious cycle of degenerating health begins, with symptoms that might take years to appear and seem intractable. These symptoms may appear in other parts of your body down the road. The treatment for them is usually to treat the consequences, not the root causes.

A brain that isn't functioning properly can help raise blood pressure as well as cause a number of digestive issues. Brain inflammation can lead to gut and joint pain as well. People might think it's just arthritis, yet arthritic lab work and x-rays are often negative. The inflammation might be arising from brain dysfunction.[1,2,3,4,5] Joint pain can be caused by brain issues. An integrated approach would also involve assisting brain function when needed.

A Healthy Gut

Bad digestion can sometimes trigger your immune system and lead to food-allergy issues. An unhealthy stomach can, among other things, create an imbalance in your gut microbial system as well as dysbiosis, which is an imbalance in the number of good and bad bacteria in your intestines.

You have more than 1,000 different types of bacteria in your intestines, and some of them are unique to you. That's why attempting to maintain gut health through a probiotics bottle isn't the complete answer, as helpful as that can be.

Are there times when eating foods and taking supplements that have the usual good nutrients can be bad for you? As with everything else related to the health of our bodies, it's not cut-and-dried.

For example, good bacteria in the wrong places in the gut can be a cause of persistent digestive problems. One example is what is called *small intestinal bacterial overgrowth,* known as SIBO. Our small intestine should have much less bacteria than our large intestine. So when the small intestine becomes populated with too much flora, or bacterial organisms, many people will feel bloated after eating meals that contain fiber, starch, and other carbohydrate products.

The excess bacteria filling the small intestine will ferment this food, creating gas and often mixed constipation or diarrhea. Fiber supplements may contribute to this problem, as they may feed the excess bacteria in the small intestine.

Foods that can exacerbate this problem include certain sugars such as fructose, starches, fiber supplements, milk from animals, many types of grains and legumes, and vegetables that we might assume would help our digestion, such as artichokes, lettuce, Brussels sprouts, and mushrooms.

If you experience a pattern of bloating after eating different types of carbohydrate-containing foods, consider that you may be suffering from SIBO.[6] Older adults in particular often have this issue, as it is the most common cause of malabsorption among older adults.[7] Since malabsorption can be an issue for many with SIBO, blood values may show signs of anemia and low protein in the serum. Low protein in the serum may in turn lead to anemia, among other problems.

People with irritable bowel syndrome and celiac disease have a much higher prevalence of SIBO. Use of proton pump inhibitors is an independent risk factor for developing SIBO. Almost all alcoholics have SIBO.[8]

A number of conditions are associated with SIBO, from thyroid issues to low stomach acid levels, immune system issues, and slow intestinal transit times, among others. Parkinson's patients often have SIBO.[9]

If you think you are having symptoms due to SIBO, consider selecting foods that do not increase fermentation in the small intestine. Constipation associated with SIBO may also be due to neurological issues and should be checked.

There are food plans on the Internet for SIBO that have helped many people. Stanford University offers a free food plan, the Low FODMAP Diet (http://fodmapliving.com/the-science/stanford-university-low-fodmap-diet/). This diet has also worked well for many people with irritable bowel syndrome and inflammatory bowel disease.

A lot of people who think they have gluten sensitivity may have SIBO instead.[10]

Those who had irritable bowel syndrome and went on a FODMAP diet had fewer intestinal issues, according to research, than those who remained on the standard dietary plan for irritable bowel syndrome.[11,12]

Some people diagnosed with irritable bowel syndrome may, in addition, be suffering from problems absorbing fructose or glucose. If you go on the Low FODMAP diet and still have issues, try eliminating fructose and glucose for a month and see how you feel.

Fiber is an essential part of maintaining good intestinal flora, yet Americans eat less than half of the recommended amount, around 30 grams a day. Obese people eat less fiber than individuals with normal weight or overweight people. Fiber intake has shown to be helpful in decreasing appetite and lowering blood sugar levels.

Gut health is important for a number of reasons. Having the wrong types and amounts of microbes can cause you to gain weight more easily because of the way they metabolize food. But the right type can help protect you against food allergies.[13]

The wrong microbes can increase your appetite level. Additionally, changes in the intestines' share of the trillions of bugs that live in our bodies, known as the *microbiome,* can increase one's chances of developing type 1 diabetes.

A study showed that infants who were predisposed through their genes to type 1 diabetes experienced a 25 percent drop in the diversity of microbes in their gut, especially the beneficial microbes, one year before developing the disease.[14] When mice with the equivalent of type 1 diabetes, which is an autoimmune disease, had their intestinal microbes transferred to mice without the disease, the mice that received the transfer showed an increased prevalence of diabetes.[15]

This evidence helps to teach us the intricately interwoven way that our body works, in this case intestinal inflammation leading to a propensity to develop type 1 diabetes. It is observed over and over in the ways that systems of our body help heal, or harm, other systems.[16]

The bacteria found in your intestines constitute about three pounds of your overall weight. Yes, there are trillions of them, right now, inside of you, perhaps as many as 100 trillion.

They are there usually either helping or hurting you. A disruption in this gut microbial balance, or dysbiosis, can accelerate a common liver condition known as *fatty liver*, which can lead to a more serious inflammation that can in turn lead to liver cancer.[17,18]

This imbalance of bacteria has been shown to increase blood sugar levels, cholesterol, and triglycerides, among other things. It can also reduce levels of B vitamins, zinc, and magnesium, which over time can lead to other symptoms.[19,20,21,22]

With this in mind, let's explore another connection between our digestive system and our brain, Alzheimer's disease.

Low levels of zinc have important effects on our health. Zinc is the most abundant trace mineral in our brain; however, those suffering from Alzheimer's have lower levels of zinc. Six months of zinc supplementation has been shown in one research study to provide significant benefits to the function of the brain for memory and reasoning.[23,24] Prolonged use of antacids decreases the absorption of dietary zinc.

Here's another example of how the body is connected in ways unexpected but important.

It turns out that when gastric bypass surgeries were first performed, surgeons noticed an unexpected beneficial side effect. High blood sugar levels were lowered for many patients. Remember that we talked about the benefits of good bacteria in the gut? Researchers found that a big reason why people lost weight wasn't just because of the intended long-term effect of decreased nutrient intake and absorption in the small intestine. The surgery was having an effect on certain cell receptors and microbes in the gut. This helped bring the patients' weight down, as well as their high sugar levels.[25,26]

The composition of the bacteria in your gut has a strong effect on how much your sugar levels rise after meals, even if you eat "bad foods"! When you increase the good levels of healthy bacteria and lower levels of the unhealthy ones, your sugar levels after eating don't increase as much.[27] That's important because higher postprandial glucose responses are associated with a higher incidence of metabolic syndrome, hypertension, cardiovascular disease, and diabetes.[28]

Systems Affect Systems

The systems in our body alter our health status in a variety of ways. Researchers are now working to see if they can create the same changes with the receptors and microbes in the intestines without having to perform stomach-reducing surgery.[29] This also shows us why it's important to keep a clinical eye on the body's entire functional status to help with a particular condition, and not just decrease symptom levels.

How your brain works, along with levels of inflammation in your body, can affect how your thyroid gland works. That can affect how well your stomach and digestive system work, as well as other systems in your body. Depression can affect how your thyroid works, which, in turn, leads to more depression.

These are examples of vicious cycles, all due to connections within our bodies that have gone largely unnoticed by a large number of clinical care providers.

It's similar to a spider web, where every strand is connected to every other strand. If you move one strand, it's felt in the entire web. At all levels, we should be looking more closely for the connections in that spider web.

Theoretical physicist Albert Einstein said that if you looked deep into nature, you would understand everything better.

In the next chapter, we will explore an example of that by examining the effects of the introduction of a wolf pack on one of America's most beloved national parks.

What You Can Do Now

- If the pain in your joints is not going away, keep in mind that brain dysfunction or intestinal issues can be a contributing cause.
- If you have bloating that goes away when you don't eat carbs, consider going on a low-FODMAP diet for a month. If the bloating ceases, you may have SIBO. If so, consider trying the Stanford University's Low FODMAP Diet.[30]

- Small-intestine issues have been linked to Parkinson's, alcoholism, and gluten sensitivities. A trial of FODMAP dieting may provide relief in ways unexpected.

- Alzheimer's has been associated with low zinc levels in the brain. Supplementation with zinc has shown to be of benefit. Proton pump inhibitors, such as Nexium, Prilosec, and Omeprazole, among others, can interfere with zinc absorption.

[16]

Wolves and the Big Picture

LET'S TAKE A look at some more practical examples of how this important pattern, this interconnection within our body, affects our well-being.

If you were a physician and had a patient with eye problems, you might approach the problem as Chinese-medicine practitioners have done for thousands of years.

In cases involving eye problems, Chinese physicians have often looked at the liver for the origin of the problem. They believe that both are connected and that when the liver is not functioning properly, eye problems can result. Western medicine now has research showing a correlation between liver function and eye problems.[1,2,3,4]

Another example that highlights this connection is the way in which our body interacts with our thoughts.

Research shows that people who suppress emotions have higher incidences of chronic lower back pain. In one study, the researchers found that San Francisco municipal bus drivers who suppressed their emotions, more than other drivers, experienced more frequent bouts of lower back pain.[5]

Next time a bus driver snaps at you, well, you can at least take comfort in knowing that you are helping him to keep his low pain from recurring!

In fact, our mind can play as important a role in the development of chronic lower back pain as biomedical issues.[6,7,8,9] The extent of childhood psychological trauma strongly affected whether lower back surgery would be successful in a retrospective study involving 86 patients.[10,11] Another study, this one involving 101 patients, indicated that chronic lower back pain, even in the absence of observable pathological structural factors, occurred more often when there were multiple psychological childhood risk factors.[12]

Childhood traumatic episodes may change the number of cell receptors in an area of our brain that is associated with fear and anxiety. This, in turn, leads to increased anxiety and reduced sociability.[13,14]

Pioneers in the clinical applications of the mind-body connection such as Bert Hellinger, Dietrich Klinghardt, Scott Walker, Donald Epstein, and Jerome Schofferman have made a point of emphasizing the hidden connections that exist between our early unresolved life experiences and present health issues.

Many ancient cultures worked with the principle that our internal states of being were root causes of health problems. In the late '90s, I had a clinic in Sardinia before moving to Rome. During lunch one day, while walking in a city on the northern part of the island, I chanced upon a museum with an exhibition of ancient Peruvian culture. There I learned that the medicine men of the Incas believed that there was one cause for all the illnesses of man. They called it "El Susto." Translated into English, it means "fear." Ancient Tibetan medicine speaks of lack of contentment as one of the principal causes of suffering and illness.

Although the phrase *mind-body connection,* and its connotations, has become well known, it's also important to keep in mind that the lesser-known *body-mind connection* also plays an important, although less well-known, part in our health.

The body-mind connection addresses the impact that our body has on our brain, how our bodies affect how we feel and express ourselves. The well-being of the tissues in our bodies, including the tone and tension of our soft tissues, is an essential part of health and of healing. There is a time-honored tradition throughout ancient and modern societies of understanding body–mind dynamics and of applying bodywork as integral to our healing.

The Complexity of Pain

"Pain is a personal experience!" I still remember one of my neurology professors driving that point home often in our classes.

He was highlighting a point that is important to anyone who suffers from chronic pain issues. As with everything else in our body, there are complexities and connections that go beyond what most consider the usual cause-and-effect cycle. Not all of our pain comes from pain receptors, known as *nociceptors,* in our body. Neurologists speak of all pain arising in our brain, not our body. How our brain processes information and how it has adapted to chronic or even acute pain can generate the experience of pain.

Regions of our brain change when we experience pain, especially chronic pain, often leading to pain being felt when there is no tissue damage. If this happens to you, the physical examination and imaging results often come back normal, and you are told that nothing is wrong or that you probably have some inflammation. Then it's off to the usual steroidal anti-inflammatory prescription.

The dynamics of chronic pain go deeper than that. The way in which our brain is wired, how it works, undergoes changes that often lead to stronger and more persistent pain. The therapies involved here that have shown success in helping people to cope with chronic pain include brain-based approaches such as tactile and motor discrimination therapies, along with operant and cognitive-based approaches.[15]

If you suffer from chronic pain, and other approaches have not been helpful, consider working with specialists in these as well as other approaches to see how training your brain can help with your pain. Free online cognitive behavior approaches have been shown to be effective in treating chronic pain, including pain associated with fibromyalgia, as well as depression and anxiety.[16,17,18]

Steroids can decrease the amount of pain by reducing inflammation. However, they do not reduce all sources of inflammation. They work primarily on prostaglandins and can have important side effects, including lowering your immune defenses.

Painkillers are generally grouped into two classes, as nonsteroidal anti-inflammatory drugs, known commonly as NSAIDs, and opioids.

NSAIDs also work by blocking prostaglandins and are also limited in how they can decrease inflammatory reactions. Using them long-term can cause intestinal damage, among other problems, because prostaglandins protect the lining of your gut.

Opioids, which include morphine, are similar to NSAIDs and steroids in that they do not block pain at the source. Opioids work by blocking pain receptors in the brain and your spinal cord. Opioids and another type of painkiller, paracetamol (acetaminophen), can also have side effects important to your health.

Now let's take a look at herbs and foods that can help with your pain. Omega-3s from fish oil, turmeric, cat's claw, devil's claw, green tea, ginger, rosemary, and willow bark have a good track record of helping with pain. So do higher levels of vitamin A and D, as well as chondroitin and glucosamine for degenerative joint conditions.

Eating alkaline foods, mentioned previously in other chapters, is also helpful.

Our body can function in a vicious cycle or a virtuous cycle, depending on how we work with it, on how we treat our body as a master gardener of health.

When we explore how our society has created health support mechanisms, we see a tendency for short-term, symptom-focused, or even illness-focused approaches, instead of approaches that look more closely at the patient as a whole.

Over half of all doctor visits are to specialists. Only one in three physicians practices in primary care.[19] However, these specialists don't often meet with the referring doctor, nor do they have conferences with other doctors to get the clinical big picture for a patient.

It does not help to minimize how useful specialists can be. We're fortunate to have them. What I am suggesting, however, is that we step back and look at the big picture of health care.

The Big Picture

I saw an interesting documentary about how Western companies took short-term approaches to profits, whereas a number of Eastern companies, from older cultures, had 50- and even 100-year goals as part of their corporate strategy. You see this short-term-focus phenomenon expressed across a number of dynamics in our culture. The way that our society approaches health care reflects this short-term approach.

Think about it: has a clinician ever sat down with you and developed a 5- or 10-year plan for your health?

Clearly, it's important not only to see the big picture but also to have the patience and discipline to make the needed changes. A healthier body needs much less discipline and effort to move in the right direction. That's important because better health means that it will be easier for you to make better lifestyle choices, including what you choose to eat.

What are some of those better choices? The more we know about the causes and effects within our bodies that are connected with our recovery and better health, the wiser our decisions. Let's take a closer look some of the ways in which cause and effect expresses itself in nature, since the dynamics of nature also apply to our health.

We know that many causes create a change in our culture and our economy. These causes can be distant and large in scope, whether it's cutting down oxygen-producing trees in the Amazon rainforest or bringing about gradual environmental changes elsewhere that cause water levels to rise. They can be physical, like an earthquake on the other side of the planet, or a shock to a stock market in another country, or a war in a small, oil-producing country thousands of miles away, creating price increases when we buy gas or related goods. But these causes can also be associated with subtle, unseen changes that can tell us more about how to view our health.

One example is the increasingly acidic ocean levels. The increased acidity is causing changes in the number and composition of phytoplanktons, which are microscopic organisms at the bottom of the seafood chain. Changes in these planktons are affecting how well the ocean absorbs carbon dioxide levels from the atmosphere.

Doesn't sound like a big deal, right?

Well, the oceans absorb approximately half of all atmospheric carbon dioxide. Those levels have been increasing for a number of years and are contributing to the greenhouse effect.

All of nature is connected in ways intricate and subtle, with significant effects on the health of the global landscape. It's the same with our bodies, with how they work and heal. Adopting an ecosystemic clinical approach would enable doctors to view and help heal their patients much more effectively.

Now, about that wolf pack, let's see how the application of this approach in a beloved national park worked out.

The history of the management of Yellowstone National Park is an interesting one. The park is different now than it was half a century ago, when the elk population was so high that the grasslands and a lot of the forests were in bad shape. Land was eroding and plants were dying off. The problem arose due to a concerted effort to kill off the wolves in the park in the early 20th century. That allowed the elk population to grow to those large numbers, since elk had been one of the wolves' chief prey animals.

After a lot of consideration, 30 wolves were reintroduced to Yellowstone in the mid-'90s. Not many wolves, really. Yet, they lowered the elk population, as intended. The funny thing is, a number of other surprising changes occurred from the introduction of just this one variable.

When the wolf population was eradicated many decades ago by the government, the local coyote population increased in large numbers. The coyotes, which had been prey of the wolves, then killed a lot of the nearby antelope. When the wolves were reintroduced in the mid-'90s, the coyote population diminished significantly, and the antelope population increased.

A much smaller number of coyotes now meant a rise in the number of their prey, such as foxes, rabbits, and young deer, as well as rodents and ground-nesting birds. Additionally, the diminished grazing by the elk and the deer allowed for more trees near the timberland to grow again. So the number of songbirds increased greatly.

Trees grew much higher in certain parts, since there were fewer elk grazing on them. That included willows, which beavers needed to get through the winter. That, in turn, allowed the number of beaver colonies to dramatically increase. Beavers were also imported and could now thrive in better conditions.

The beavers helped to recharge the water table and provide shading for fish, as well as a way to stabilize water runoff. The dams that the beavers constructed helped to stop erosion and created ponds that fish and fowl could use. A larger number of eagles, hawks, and badgers followed—evidence of more complexity and abundance in the food chain. Then the grizzly bears found more wild fruit to eat because the overgrazing by elk herds had diminished.

When the wolves chased the deer out of certain areas of the park, a number of trees at the edge of these woods and near the riverbanks began to grow many times their previous height, helping to provide stability to the soil.[20,21,22,23]

The riverbanks stopped collapsing so often, and with fewer deer grazing, the vegetation had a chance to recover. Its roots provided stability to the soil and helped to prevent further erosion. In addition, the greater number of beavers also helped to diminish erosion.

A lot of damage had already been done by the elk through the decades, so the effects that the wolves have had since they were reintroduced are still limited, but noticeable.

Wolves had an effect on changing the courses of rivers . . . and a lot more!

Many of these problems were symptoms of a lack of ecological balance due to how the park administrators managed the park in the early 20th century, similar to how much of medicine continues to be practiced.

Rather than simply continuing to replant trees or using sandbags to stabilize the erosion in the riverbanks, the rangers now saw things differently. They saw a bigger picture. They studied what might be a root cause and what could bring back a number of needed changes, in a natural way.

They reintroduced wolves into the environment and brought back more balance to the ecosystem. Now Yellowstone has more tools to self-regulate in a healthier way.

There's a striking parallel between this story and your body's ability to self-regulate and heal, reminding us that in order to find and address the underlying barriers to healing, we must first look for the root causes, for the subtle connections that can make a big difference.

Hidden Anemia Connections

How would this specifically relate to someone's health challenge? Let's explore a condition that is associated with feeling tired and is so common that half of all nursing-home residents have it—anemia.

Many patients are given iron tablets for anemia. For a number of them, it has been shown that these tablets don't consistently raise iron levels. People with anemia can feel cold and complain that their brain doesn't function well.

Lack of iron is the most common cause of anemia, but not the only one. An important question to ask is what is chronically causing low iron levels in a number of patients, even though they have been prescribed iron supplements for many years?

It's similar to repeatedly planting seedlings because the elk have been eating the leaves, but not looking at the root causes, not addressing the elk overpopulation.

You may remember that we have already discussed why someone might not be absorbing iron, especially among the elderly. Low stomach acid levels, as well as intestinal problems, could contribute to a person's not absorbing minerals well, including iron. As we grow older, our bodies produce less of the needed acid, making it more difficult for us to absorb a number of minerals, including iron.

Calcium and copper are also needed to help the body assimilate iron. There might be other reasons for low blood iron levels, such as heavy menstruation patterns in cycling women or intestinal bleeding, among others.

When we help people with this type of chronic problem by giving them digestive aids to support the function and health of their stomach and intestines, many times we see this issue begin to clear up. Iron levels measured by blood tests start to rise, and anemia markers associated with low iron start to normalize, often for the first time in years. People then feel better and less tired.

Sometimes the most important thing you can do to help your chronic health issues is to . . . find your wolf pack!

What You Can Do Now

- Consider aiding the liver's function to address eye issues. Supporting liver function may help support eye health. A number of supplements, including milk thistle and dandelion tea, nutritionally support liver function.

- Consider addressing how you handle emotions if you are suffering from chronic low back pain, or other issues, and have difficulty expressing your emotions. Counseling and therapy can help where biomedical approaches have failed, especially if there are unresolved painful childhood events.

- Behavioral and cognitive therapies are known to address pain successfully. Free online cognitive behavioral approaches are now available that research has shown to work well. They have also been proven effective at dealing with anxiety and depression. One well-known site, from Australia, is MoodGYM (https://moodgym.anu.edu.au/welcome). A website that is geared for children is Biteback (http://www.biteback.org.au/).

- Iron pills are not a panacea for chronic anemia. Look for root causes, including digestive issues leading to malabsorption, or other causes. The elderly usually have low levels of hydrochloric acid, which affects the ability to assimilate a number of minerals and other nutrients.

[17]
All for One

IF WE TURN on the news, we quickly see how connected and interdependent things are around the world. We're becoming more aware, through technology, of this connection, of this interrelationship.

It will benefit us if our society views and provides health care the same way that the good people at Yellowstone National Park have managed it, and adapt more integrated approaches to reveal more root causes and more issues that are contributing to our illnesses.

The good news is, all that's required to get a really good start in that direction is to change how we see things.

The bad news, unfortunately, is that changing viewpoints and opinions is one of the hardest things to do. Often, money and energy go into more technological advances rather than changing paradigms in clinical approaches, of seeing the usual differently.

For instance, when doctors think it's necessary, they send you to a specialist and wait for a report to come back. If you have a thyroid issue and heart palpitations, and they think the heart should be checked, they might wisely send you to a second specialist. If you also have a recurring digestive issue, the doctor might send you to yet another specialist somewhere else, who typically will run some lab and diagnostic tests, and then your doctor will wait for that specialist's report.

How often have you been in a room when all your specialists were there at one time, or even on a brief telephone conference call? Doing so would give you the benefit of having your doctors confer with one another and offer clinical insights to your primary treating physician.

Most patients don't have the advantage of this health situation room, of knowing that meetings are taking place between the specialists involved with their health place to ensure that the clinical choices made are the best ones for them.

Obviously that's not feasible on routine visits, but we have missed the clinical boat often enough by using a segregated, sectional clinical approach. I am suggesting that we look at the benefits of an integrated, interconnected clinical philosophy that includes physicians actively conferring with each other to look for more causative or contributive factors to health concerns. Clinicians would be actively involved in care coordination at an expanded level and from different healing approaches.

Most people spend only a few minutes with their doctors. A lot of doctors are frustrated about this and would like to spend more time with each patient, but the present system is not set up that way.

At an individual level, a doctor's greatest ability to help a patient as a whole is to step back and consider the bigger clinical picture, and to look for seemingly unrelated clinical clues.

We live in an age of growing medical specialization. Specialists have been described as those knowing more and more about less and less. That is not meant to denigrate or minimize their place and importance.

However, there is a strong emphasis on continuing to rely on Cartesian-based clinical paradigms, a rationalistic approach that has as its clinical equivalent looking through more and more powerful microscopes to determine what's wrong with the patient.

While it is useful, we need to include the appropriate equivalency of clinical telescopes—a wide-view, big-picture approach to best help a patient to heal more fully. It calls for a balanced use of deductive as well as inductive reasoning.

We want to be in a position to have the best of both worlds: the modernity of technology merged with the antiquity of wisdom. I speak of the wisdom of older societies that reflected deep insights into the workings of nature, which they depended on every day for their survival—and health.

It's fundamental for us as clinicians to inquire into what we can do for the patient to help facilitate these interconnected, self-healing mechanisms of the body. These mechanisms depend on the entire body working at its best to support your better health.

We've discussed how lab work is a very limited indicator of whole body function. Many times you can have a normally functioning organ or system that may need to work harder to provide support to another part of the body that is in distress or in illness. Lab or imaging tests for these situations only show signs when the body has reached the red-light level.

Common sense tells us, however, that it's the common-sense thing for the body to do. Remember the last time you moved? If you have four people carrying a heavy sofa, and let's say one of them starts to feel pain and is unable to continue lifting equally, then the others will have to strain to keep carrying the sofa. I have highlighted many instances throughout this book where failing or suboptimal body parts have impacted others negatively.

Our health system is not set up to take notice of subclinical compensations that other parts of the body need to do to help us become healthier, especially for chronic issues. A typical response is that the usual physical exam and lab work show no issues. Yet, as was noted in an earlier chapter, by the time a lab result comes back as abnormal, you have slipped into the last 5 percent of an unhealthy population group.

In the previous chapter, I mentioned the Chinese medicine view of the liver and the eyes as one example of how other healing approaches look at other parts of the body to help one in obvious distress to work better. Here's another example. The kidneys filter and excrete many of the toxins metabolized by the liver. If the liver is not working well, the kidneys may feel the strain of more metabolized toxins than usual running through it. From a holistic perspective, it would be wise to consider natural support for the kidneys, even if the blood workup returns normal. For many, research shows that the single most important thing people can do to help their body work better is to lose weight.

For most, that's not easy. But, fortunately, it can be.

Let's find out how.

What You Can Do Now

- When you have complex health problems and have been sent from specialist to specialist with little improvement, ask your primary treating physician if it's possible for them to talk together. More and more hospitals and clinics are doing this, as they have found that sharing and integrating their insights creates greater benefits for the patients.
- Consider natural aids, such as food, herbs, and other therapies, that could be useful to support organ and

tissue function. For information on herbs, some of which may be contraindicated in some conditions or while taking certain drugs, the University of Maryland has a website with more information (https://umm.edu/health/medical/altmed/treatment/herbal-medicine).

- The American Herbalist Guild also has more information (http://www.americanherbalistguild.com).

[18]

How to Make the Weight Slide Right Off

I TELL PEOPLE, because I see it a number of times each day in my clinic, that weight loss can happen quite easily for many people while experiencing good energy levels and no hunger. It should not be a period of suffering or strain. In fact, that's a prerequisite to losing weight in our clinic: feeling good.

As your body heals, you'll find it easier to make healthier food choices. Numerous patients come in stating that they have a strong craving for sugar products or breads. Later, as their body heals, they tell me with surprise, and relief, that while they still enjoy these foods, they no longer feel such a strong attraction to eating them.

They find themselves eating smaller amounts of food and making healthier choices, without having to be disciplined about it. Many people whose bodies don't work well and feel tired, start off by trying to lose weight. Their bodies aren't ready for it. It's like putting the cart in front of the horse.

A lot of patients tell me that they seem to have lost more weight around their belly than what the loss on their bathroom scale would typically indicate. I let them know that this is actually a good thing!

I rarely tell patients to limit their meal portions, because most of them find that their natural appetite level returns in a way that helps them drop excess weight. The key is to be healthy enough so that your body can more easily support a weight-loss regimen. This also helps to keep the weight loss stable.

This is the general health approach that we have been discussing: looking at your body and your health from a larger perspective. It also applies to losing fat.

Every person is unique, our bodies are different from one another's, and each person has undergone life experiences and challenges that are unique to him or her, so that each clinical approach, or weight-loss program, needs to be tailored individually.

Therefore, why should everyone be on the same diet or exercise program, or on the same pills, even if they are touted as natural?

People of one body type might find it easier to lose weight and to feel better eating foods that are quite different from those preferred by people of other body types. This also applies to the timing of the foods eaten.

When it comes to taking care of your health, either for weight loss or for a set of conditions, the best place to start is with an examination approach that takes you, as well as your issues, into account. This could include blood tests, stool tests, hormone tests, urine tests, and other types of screening tests as needed, including genetic testing, to help develop the best clinical approach for every individual. Later in the book we will discuss in more detail how individually designed nutrition programs that are based on a number of your unique clinical parameters, including gut microbial testing, will become commonplace in clinical nutrition strategies.

Food, exercise, lifestyle, and supplements when necessary are basic ground-floor approaches. There are also times when it's best to refer the patient to another doctor who is in a more appropriate branch of the healing arts, and to work together as a team.

We live in a culture of abundance, and we tend to project that onto our approach to health and weight loss. If some things are good, why not take a bunch of them? We continue taking hundreds of supplements throughout the years, and keep buying the next new miracle pill, machine, or vitamin product that's supposed to cure this or that—and it's not as if they don't have a place when necessary.

Your small intestines, which are where most of the nutrients in your food are absorbed, have a limited amount of foods/vitamins/supplements that they can actually use. Given the limitations of your digestive system, choose with discretion what nutritional support you want to emphasize, in order to get the most out of it.

However, when your body is healthy enough on the inside, when you sleep well and have naturally good energy levels, and the systems in your body are working better, then your desire for junk food slips into the background.

We've been taught in books and magazines, on TV and radio shows, as well as during doctor visits, what to eat and what not to eat. By now, many people don't need someone to sit down behind a desk and tell them how to do that again. For most, it's just that their body is not ready to cooperate. Emotional eating, among other things, is harder to control in an unhealthy body.

I was talking to Tina, a patient who, after years of frustration and doubts about her self-discipline, had increased her energy and well-being while losing weight.

She shared with me how much stress she felt particularly about her extended hours at work, as well as her favorite comfort food. Here's what she said: "In the past, it was a lot easier to stuff myself or dig through a pint of ice cream. I still love the taste of ice cream and eat it from time to time, but it doesn't feel like a compulsion. So the choice is a lot easier now. I still feel some urges when someone at work or at home upsets me, but it's just easier now to make better choices."

Emotional eating is a challenge for many, one that goes beyond self-discipline. If a person is in a negative emotional state, the taste of foods actually changes. Healthy food, such as vegetables, will not taste as good as usual, while the attraction to sweets, and the pleasure of their taste, increases.[1]

To help reach the body shape we'd like to be in and to make it easier to make healthier food choices, let's explore what sick dogs can teach us about weight loss, and more!

What You Can Do Now

- What works for one person for weight loss may not work for you. Look for a program that best fits your needs. A clinical program that helps you to successfully and more easily lose weight starts by helping your body to become healthier.
- Body dysfunction makes it harder for any food plan to work well. When you start feeling better, you will start making better food choices. Hang in there, and put a particular emphasis on healing any sleep and low-energy issues.
- If you had a bad food choice day, consider writing briefly in a journal that night how you were feeling during the day. Then write just a couple of lines at the end on ways that you could have responded differently with your food choices.

- Reread the journal periodically to help you see your responses with more perspective. It won't change the calorie count of the day that just passed, but it can help you to express and release some emotional patterns that could enable you to make better choices the next time a similar dynamic comes around . . . and life has a way of bringing back patterns, often until we develop better ways of handling them!

[19]

A Sick Dog's Weight-Loss Lessons

HAVE YOU EVER noticed that when a dog is sick, it eats grass, more so than usual?

The reasons why they do that are not fully known. Grass is not a source of nutrition for them, however, and when this happens, a veterinarian might suggest that you bring your dog in to see if it's ill. When the dog is healthy again, it usually stops eating grass or eats it a lot less.

Ask yourself, if dogs eat grass when they are feeling ill, what do sick people eat when they feel ill, or are simply not in good health?

When people aren't healthy, they tend to eat unhealthy food, just like a sick dog. When people are feeling healthier, more rested, and more energetic, and the cells of their bodies are communicating and working well, they start eating better and putting the unhealthy food to the side. Making the choice to eat healthier foods arises out of a healthier body.

Most people who want to lose weight put the cart in front of the horse.

Have you ever asked yourself why we think about weight loss the way we do? We treat weight loss the way health issues are usually treated: by focusing on the symptom—the consequence, and not its root causes. Think of a sick dog eating grass, and ask yourself, what inside of you is driving you to eat the way you do?

What connections within your body do you need to be aware of?

Obesity as a Symptom

Let's think for the time being of weight gain as a symptom, a consequence, while acknowledging that a condition like obesity has far-ranging health implications. A symptom arising from some sources can also be a cause for other problems.

Each year, an estimated 300,000 adults in the U.S. die of causes related to obesity.[1] To put it into perspective, complications arising from obesity kill a population the size of Pittsburgh, Pennsylvania, year after year.

Obesity also has an effect on your brain as you get older. There is an association between being more overweight at age 50 and a quicker onset of Alzheimer's, for those who develop it. For every increased unit of body mass index, or BMI, which is an approximate measure of your body fat based on height-to-weight levels, earlier onset of Alzheimer's increases by almost seven months. That risk factor does not change even if you are keeping your cardiovascular system in shape through exercise. Additionally, the greater your BMI at the age of 50, the greater the amount of brain damage associated with Alzheimer's upon autopsy.[2]

Knowing something like that, would you want to address a symptom by treating only the symptom itself or, as we have been exploring throughout this book, look for the root issues that caused or contributed to the symptom?

Most people don't think of excess weight as a symptom, only that they are getting fat and don't like the tight-fitting jeans and bulging stomachs. The problem with being overweight extends much further than perhaps you or someone you know—or even the country. It's a worldwide problem.

Many think that obesity problems are primarily confined to the United States and a few other countries, the ones with a fast-food place located every few blocks. Unfortunately, they're not.[3] There are now more than two billion people who are either obese or overweight. Almost a third of the world is fat.

An international study was conducted on weight loss that spanned more than three decades. Guess how many of the 188 countries that were studied over a period of 33 years had a significant decline in obesity during that time?

Given all the popular weight-loss programs out there, the books, the talk shows, the new diets, and the research that has come out about eating well and exercising, one would think that the more educated nations, such as the United States, would have seen a strong reduction.

Unfortunately, none of the 188 countries experienced a significant decline in obesity—despite all the information, all the new research on eating well, and all those great diets, TV shows, websites, and books.[4]

The approaches being used today are obviously not working.

Diets can help people lose weight in the short term, but research reveals that they are not making a dent when you look at the larger picture. These statistics show that the challenges and frustrations that you or others might have been feeling for a number of years in the struggle to lose weight are being experienced worldwide.

In a 13-year period recently studied, after adjusting for age, Americans' waistlines expanded by more than one inch. The majority of people now have abdominal obesity.[5]

DIABETES

To complicate things, at the rate we have been going, 40 percent of adults in the United States will develop diabetes in this lifetime due to being overweight or obese. Two million Americans are diagnosed with diabetes each year. That number jumps to 50 percent of adults for Hispanics.

It's bad news for a number of reasons. For example, one of the little-known connections associated with diabetes is that middle-aged diabetics have a greater chance of developing cognitive decline, such as Alzheimer's, by the time they reach 70.[6]

These rates of increase in mental dysfunction apply to prediabetics as well, including those with blood sugar levels around 110 and higher.

Diabetics, as they age, lose more brain volume than nondiabetics.[7] In fact, people with diabetes have a life expectancy six years less than the average.[8]

Most diabetics die from heart disease. Half of all heart attack patients either are diabetic or have elevated blood sugar levels that are close to diabetic levels. For diabetics in particular, healthy blood pressure and cholesterol levels are important because they help reduce the risk of cardiovascular diseases.[9]

The percentage of people with diabetes in this country has almost doubled in the past 20 years. Yet some of the ways to help prevent it are very simple. For example, for people with high blood sugar levels, losing 12 pounds has shown to stop the rate of progression to diabetes by 50 percent. Add moderate exercise, and the number increases to around 70 percent.[10]

Keep in mind that diabetes is not always associated with obesity. Many diabetics have normal weight. Genetics and other factors also play a role. I mentioned earlier in this book that use of prescription drugs can lead to diabetes, noting that people with normal blood sugar values who begin to take statins increase their risk of getting type 2 diabetes by two and a half times.

Another factor that influences rates of type 2 diabetes significantly is where your calories come from. The conventional wisdom is to focus on eating fewer calories and exercising to lose weight and reduce the incidence of diabetes. There is obviously truth to this line of thought; however, a connection exists between the type of calories and the rate of diabetes that most people are not aware of.

Many people think it's OK to eat sugary food as long as they do enough exercise to burn it off. Unfortunately, there is a hidden connection, one most are not aware of, that limits the ability of exercise to counteract how that junk food will affect you. As you have already read, the body's complex set of processes works beyond the simple mechanistic approach of eating calories and working out to burn them off.

Exercising on a regular basis has wonderful benefits, but it does not erase all the effects of bad food habits. Every 150 calories of sugar that you ingest in excess of the maximum that a person should consume—for example, what you would drink in a typical can of soda—leads to an 11-fold increase in the prevalence of type 2 diabetes when compared with the same 150 excess calories ingested from protein or fat. That happens regardless of your level of activity.[11,12]

This dramatic spike in the prevalence of diabetes also occurs regardless of your weight.[13,14] Almost half of children who are considered to have a normal body mass index will have health issues that can include high cholesterol, cardiovascular diseases, high blood pressure, and liver diseases.[15]

The quality of the food you eat, and not just the calories, makes a big hidden impact on health challenges that are normally associated with obesity.

It's self-evident that not all calories are created equal!

Weight loss is obviously important, yet it needs to be looked at differently, so let's put our attention on some common eating habits that are the result of poor health.

Many patients tell me that they usually crave sweets between meals and usually feel a lot better after they eat them. Others say that they get irritable when they miss a meal, tire easily, and have difficulty staying asleep.

Many report that for a number of years they have been suffering from chronic stress and have been feeling lower energy levels. Almost half of all adults don't think they are managing stress well.

Research shows that there is a connection between these symptoms, emotional eating patterns, and expanding love handles, those fat bulges around the waist.[16]

Cortisol

When people have been under stress for years, it puts a lot of pressure on the body's stress-response system. When stress occurs, whether emotional or due to a problem with your body, your adrenal glands, which are two small glands that sit on top of your kidneys, create a hormone called *cortisol*.

Cortisol is a stress-response hormone that also has anti-inflammatory properties, along with many other effects in your body. When you are under stress for long periods of time, your adrenal glands can get tired of producing this hormone and will start to produce less.

But before the adrenals get tired of producing cortisol, they have usually been pumping out a lot of cortisol in response to your stress for many years. Often the rhythm of this cortisol release, controlled by the brain, is also altered, causing a number of issues.

Over time, this can have a lot of negative effects on your body. The cause of the production of chronic high cortisol levels is not limited to emotional stress. It can be from physical stress, nutritional issues, insulin resistance, chronic infections, brain dysfunction, and environmental stress.

One of the many functions of cortisol is that it helps increase blood sugar levels in between meals so that you have a more stable sugar level. The pancreas produces the hormone *glucagon* to help balance blood sugar levels. *Adrenaline* is another hormone produced by the adrenal glands to help your body put sugar in your blood for use by your body.

Why do so many people have hunger pangs between meals that can only be satisfied by eating high-carb food?

Well, one reason is that the adrenal output over time becomes sluggish and the glands don't produce enough cortisol between meals, which can lead to sugar levels dropping. That, in turn, can make people hungry for sweets.

You can get these sweet cravings because the body, especially your brain, needs sugar; in fact, a part of your brain activates hunger when blood levels drop.

These sugar cravings are often associated with irritability and complaining of not thinking very well, or of occasional blurred vision. That's because the body and brain are low on fuel. Another reason is that if you don't have enough carbs to stimulate a strong enough insulin response after a meal, the receptors in your hypothalamus, that part of your brain that helps to regulate your appetite, are not activated sufficiently to produce a sense of being satisfied with what you ate. There are more biochemicals produced in your body to also help regulate your appetite.

The complexity of interaction within our body systems also applies to something as apparently simple as feeling satisfied and full after a meal!

Serotonin and Weight

This is a good time to bring up the subject of neurotransmitters, because they are a major player in the eating habits of most people. Among other things, neurotransmitters are chemical messengers, some of which are responsible for how well you feel, such as serotonin. Hormones are also chemical messengers, but usually larger in size.

I mentioned before that low serotonin levels are traditionally associated with depression, although recent studies have revealed that the issue is more complex and needs more study.

Low serotonin levels are also associated with a number of other issues, including autism.

But let's focus on this neurotransmitter as it relates to eating and weight issues. Serotonin is affected by a number of things, including low blood sugar, known as *hypoglycemia*. Low blood sugar also affects memory, concentration, and reasoning. Adequate levels of serotonin in your brain help you to eat less.

People commonly think that serotonin is made only in the brain. In fact, almost all of your body's serotonin is made in your gut and helps to control the rate of bowel movements. It's not the only thing that serotonin does. The emerging field of neurogastroenterology is studying how the network of neurons in the walls of your intestines, which is known as the enteric system, can affect mood and a number of diseases. In fact, they have a term for this part of the nervous system that has more neurons than the spinal cord: the *second brain*.

Serotonin is associated with feelings of well-being and relaxation. One reason why many people have a craving for carbohydrate-rich meals, especially simple carbs, is because the insulin that is produced by the body after you eat carbs helps the brain to produce higher levels of serotonin, making you feel better.

It sounds like, and is, a barrier to losing weight. You don't feel good, so you instinctively eat some high-calorie foods, simple carbohydrates, often a lot of them, and feel better. However, there is a way that you can use this to your advantage and not let it continue to sabotage so many of your well-meaning attempts to lose weight!

Now that you know about this connection between increased serotonin levels, feeling good, and food, let's use it to help you lose weight.

When your emotions are leading you to eat this way, knowing that low brain serotonin levels are usually involved, have a snack, but limit yourself to around 20 grams of carbohydrates, preferably simple carbs, like a cracker or a cookie that has around 80 calories.

That is enough to trigger a series of processes in your body that will boost your serotonin levels in a short period of time, helping you to feel better, yet it makes a small dent in your total daily calorie intake!

Your brain weighs about three pounds but accounts for about 20 percent of your entire body's glucose, or sugar, requirements.[17] Glucose is the brain's main fuel source. So low blood sugar affects brain function. A lot of people who don't feel well say that they feel better when they snack on potato chips, cookies, or other high-carbohydrate foods.

Low serotonin levels can be an issue, but so can low blood sugar levels. To understand more about junk-food cravings, we will explore the connections between low blood sugar and a couple of small but important glands in your body.

The Adrenal Glands

When the brain is not working well, people tend to make bad decisions more often, including decisions about food.

For many, frequent cravings for sugar and other refined carbs are the result of low-functioning adrenals. They have been overworked for years due to chronic high levels of stress. This is one reason why many people find it difficult to lose weight. It's not the only reason for these types of cravings, but with our bodies being as complex as they are, it's usually the case. Among other things, deficiencies in minerals, such as chromium, can also affect sugar cravings.

Many people try to balance these cravings, or try to decrease the number of calories they eat, by using artificial sweeteners.

Artificial sweeteners, however, have been shown to increase blood sugar levels as well, which can lead to diabetes. They do so by altering the bacteria in your gut.[18] In a study involving older people, drinking diet sodas on a regular basis was shown to have a direct association with increasing the waist sizes of adults 65 years and older.[19]

I've mentioned that low blood sugar and fatigue are often associated with the adrenal glands. The adrenal glands help provide your body with energy and produce anti-inflammatory substances such as cortisol. They also perform a lot of other functions, such as creating other hormones and helping stabilize fluid levels.

Like every process in the body, good adrenal function depends on a number of things, including nutrition, such as an adequate level of vitamin C.

The adrenals have one of the highest rates of storage of vitamin C content of any part of your body. Vitamin C is water-soluble, which means that it can be used up more quickly during stress.

Low levels can affect adrenal function. When your adrenal glands secrete cortisol to fight inflammation or stress, they also secrete vitamin C, causing your body to need more of it.[20]

If you are under a lot of stress, emotional or physical, especially if it has been going on for a long time, consider taking in more vitamin C. Do so not only for its antioxidant abilities, but because it will help to shore up your adrenals, which in turn may help to decrease your sugar cravings.

Certain centers in the brain send information to the adrenals to regulate the volume and frequency of needed hormones. If your adrenal glands are not working well, it could create a low blood sugar situation that could affect the working of your brain, which in turn helps regulate adrenal function.

This can create a physiological vicious cycle that impairs the sincere efforts of many people caught in the cycle to lose weight. My motto is: Focus on your health first; then weight loss will follow more easily.

In other words, fix the body to fix the fat!

Many people suffer from this and a number of other issues in their body at the same time. That's why a symptom-based, one-pill approach, even if using supplements or herbs, usually won't end this vicious cycle.

Another factor of obesity involves a person's sleep patterns. It has been shown that people who don't sleep well tend to overeat on those days.[21]

This leads to our next question: Can your adrenals, those glands that help you to respond to stress, also have an effect on sleep issues?

What You Can Do Now

- Don't wait until you are diagnosed with diabetes to take strong action to lower your blood sugar levels. Among the elderly, pre-diabetics experience the same greater rates of mental dysfunction as diabetics.
- A few pounds do matter. Even dropping 10 pounds or so can significantly slow the progression toward diabetes.
- It's not just the number of calories but also the type of calories you end up consuming that can significantly increase your risk of diabetes. On that issue, if you are going to overeat, consider going more for protein than refined carbs, especially if there is a family history of diabetes.
- Sugar cravings, especially between meals, may mean that you could benefit from mid-meal protein snacks

to help regulate blood sugar levels. And consider vitamin C supplementation as well as natural aids for better adrenal function.

- Stress has you opening your kitchen cabinets? Eat just a little bit of a cracker or bread, enough to help your brain make more serotonin and take the emotional edge off.

- Sleepless in Seattle? See above. Eating a cracker before going to bed can help your brain make more melatonin, since melatonin is made from serotonin. I have a patient who finds that this is the only way she can go to sleep.

[20]

Obesity and Inflammation: A Terrible Twosome

MOST OF OUR chronic diseases have their roots in inflammation. Obesity is a low-grade inflammatory condition. Fat tissues stimulate the production of inflammatory compounds in our body. Obesity is associated with an increased risk of several types of cancer, such as endometrial and colon cancers. There are also connections between obesity, being a postmenopausal woman, and breast cancer.

The majority of breast cancers in postmenopausal women are the estrogen-receptor positive types. Even though the ovaries of postmenopausal women have ceased to produce estrogen, fat tissues continue to produce it. The more fat, or adipose tissue, that a woman has, the greater the production of estrogen in her body, including an increase in estrogen generated by her breast fat. In overweight or obese women, that increases the risk of having this type of breast cancer.[1]

Could there be a connection between overeating and inflammation in our bodies?

You bet your large bag of salty chips there is. Research is showing that gut bacteria issues, which can lead to low-grade inflammation, are one reason why people overeat. Inflammation is not a rare thing. Looking at the gut alone, over half a million Americans have inflammatory bowel disease each year.[2]

Since not sleeping well has been shown to lead to overeating, let's look at some of the factors involved in not sleeping well. The U.S. Centers for Disease Control and Prevention (CDC) now considers insufficient sleep an epidemic.

Adrenals and Sleep

If your adrenals cannot produce enough hormones to sustain normal blood sugar levels between meals, guess what happens a few hours after you go to sleep?

A lot of people will end up waking up two or three hours after they go to sleep and then have a hard time going back to sleep again. They start going over events of the day, and they toss and turn, thinking that anxiety is keeping them from returning to sleep. Then they tell their doctor about this issue, and the doctor may end up prescribing something for what is thought to be a problem arising from anxiety.

But this sleep loss might not be an emotional issue. In fact, it can be associated with sugar cravings, which is a consequence—not the primary problem. I mentioned that not sleeping well leads people to eat more throughout the day.

The brain uses glucose, or blood sugar, as its favorite form of fuel. We have talked about cortisol helping the body, through the liver, to maintain enough blood sugar available for the brain, which is quite active at night. Some of the natural support that you can use to help stabilize your cortisol levels at night and help you to improve your sleep quality include eating a few pieces of licorice a day, and eating cinnamon in the evening. Tomatoes can also help with sleep by increasing melatonin, which is a hormone that promotes sleep.

If the adrenal glands do not secrete enough cortisol to help stabilize blood sugar levels, the body responds by creating another stress hormone, a strong, immediate-stress hormone that I mentioned earlier—adrenaline.

Think of it as a "super" hormone. It's the body's urgent way of getting sugar into your blood right then and there. It does other things as well; for instance, it puts needed sugar into your blood for the brain to use. But since it is an emergency hormone, it wakes you up and makes it harder for you to go back to sleep.

This is one way that sugar cravings during the day can be connected to a low-functioning adrenal gland, which can lead to dysfunctional sleeping patterns. This might not always be the cause, but we often see this type of sleep dysfunction with patients. There are variations and other dynamics that can take place. For example, *hyperarousal* is a term used to describe increased brain activity at night and is clinically associated with insomnia. Increased activity can happen in one or in various parts of the brain simultaneously. Dysregulation of the area of the brain commonly associated with memory, the hippocampus, as well as disruptions in the HPA axis, known as the *hypothalamic-pituitary-adrenal axis,* are common. In turn, they can lead to disruptions in the proper levels and timing of cortisol and have been associated with hyperarousal.

Stress and Cortisol

When we are stressed out for long periods of time, the body creates a chronically elevated level of cortisol, which can eventually cause our adrenal glands to decrease their output, producing lower levels of cortisol than normal.

Some people's adrenal glands seem to tire out more quickly than others; some have strong glands that can produce for years or decades, or even a lifetime. And some people start feeling the effects much earlier, even in their youth.

There has been some controversy regarding the term *adrenal fatigue.* Some clinicians feel that the correct term is *adrenal insufficiency,* which is usually associated with an autoimmune disease and sharply reduced adrenal hormone levels.

However, research shows that chronic stress can lead to a reduction in cortisol levels over time, as the adrenals initially pump out a higher amount at the beginning of a stressful event and then a lesser amount as the stress responses continue over a longer period of time. Adrenal glands enlarge when they are under chronic stress.[3,4,5,6,7,8] We will discuss that in more depth later.

Chronically high cortisol levels also affect calcium absorption in the intestines; can reduce bone formation, leading to osteoporosis; and can increase resistance to insulin.[9] I noted that these high levels can make it harder for you to fall asleep and that not sleeping well can raise your insulin levels, creating another vicious cycle while stimulating your appetite centers.

You can also have problems with your memory if your cortisol levels are high for too long, because this can shrink the hippocampus, which is a structure in your brain that helps with memory.[10] Ironically, the hippocampus also helps to control the rhythm of cortisol excretion.

If your hippocampus is not functioning well, in turn, it can affect how well you sleep, which we mentioned can increase your weight, which also contributes to high sugar levels and brain inflammation. This can then cause harm to your hippocampus—and we are back to amplifying the effects of a vicious physiological cycle!

There's more. Emotional stress, associated with increased cortisol levels, can play an important role in the development of type 2 diabetes.[11,12]

Some people's blood sugar levels rise sharply simply because of their body's reaction to cortisol, even though they eat quite well.[13,14,15] Therefore, you can have lab-test sugar levels that are high but are not due to eating patterns or genetics—rather, these elevated levels are due to your emotions and your body's response to them.

What are some other harmful connections between your health and chronically high levels of cortisol?

Too much cortisol can increase blood pressure, affect menstrual cycles, and increase appetite, leading to weight gain.

Additionally, high levels of cortisol affect the receptors in the arcuate nucleus of the hypothalamus, the appetite/hunger center of the brain that regulates weight. That's bad news for your sustained efforts to eat well, because altered receptor function in this part of the brain can lead to increased appetite levels.[16]

What about a connection between cortisol levels and weight?

Too much cortisol over a period of time can lead to weight gain. It can also break down your body tissue and accelerate aging. It can lead to digestive problems and depression, among other symptoms.

Remember that excess cortisol makes it harder for your body to respond to the hormones that your thyroid makes? Well, cortisol will create resistance to practically all the hormones in your body. That includes female hormones and, as I mentioned, insulin.[17] Another unfortunate effect of high chronic levels of cortisol is that in making more of it, your body can reduce its sex hormone production, leading to a decreased sex drive.

It's one of the reasons why you or your partner, when under a lot of stress, can lose interest in having sex.

In addition, too much cortisol diminishes the effects of insulin injections and some other medications for those suffering from high blood sugar levels. That's why measuring cortisol levels, which can be done in a number of simple ways with lab testing, can be helpful as part of this clinical philosophy of looking at everything in the body that can be connected to your illness or condition, including indirectly.

Chronic inflammation is damaging to the body. One measure of such inflammation is the level of something called *C-reactive protein,* which is produced by the liver and blood vessels in response to inflammation in the body's inflammatory reactions. Current thinking is that C-reactive protein not only is a marker of inflammation but also contributes to inflammation.

C-reactive protein binds to *leptin,* which is the hormone that is produced by the fat cells after eating, and prevents it from crossing the blood-brain barrier to signal your brain that you have eaten enough.[18]

Obese people have higher levels of leptin in their body. Increased leptin levels are associated with higher risks of cancer.

That is one reason why some people just keep eating and eating, even after their belly is full. The body develops resistance to leptin just like it can to insulin if the levels are high for too long. When that happens, your brain does not realize that you've had enough to eat. Chronic inflammation also contributes to this. Keep in mind that you can have high levels of inflammation even if you feel no pain. Systemic inflammation is usually detected via inexpensive blood-test markers.

Posture Matters

How would you like to temporarily lower your cortisol levels in less than a couple of minutes?

Could there be a connection between higher levels of cortisol, emotions, and our posture? It turns out that slouching, whether sitting or standing, increases cortisol levels in the body. It also decreases testosterone levels and makes it easier to recall negative memories and thoughts.[19]

On the other hand, sitting or standing erect rather than slumped decreases cortisol levels, increases testosterone levels, and makes it easier to recall uplifting memories and thoughts. The change in memory patterns, sense of energy, and hormone levels can occur in less than two minutes when you change your posture.[20,21,22] You can watch a 30-second video by NOVA on YouTube by one of the researchers. It teaches a power pose that creates those types of changes for you. The video's title is: *Amy Cuddy: 30 Seconds on Power Poses.*

Your mother's advice to stop slouching actually has scientific merit!

Decreasing Inflammation

Let's look at foods that help decrease inflammation, which would also help bring chronic cortisol levels down. Eating less red meat or trying to eliminate it completely would be helpful. Also, consider regularly exercising, reducing or eliminating alcohol and caffeine, eating healthy foods, and reducing or eliminating excessive acid-producing foods, such as breads, sugar products, and refined carbohydrates.

Fasting; high-intensity exercise; and *ketogenic* diets, commonly known as fat-burning diets, have been shown to decrease inflammation by creating a compound that helps to lower inflammatory processes in the body.

If you are still wondering if inflammation is really that big a deal for you, especially if you don't feel inflamed, know that chronic inflammation is also associated with many diseases, including diabetes, autoimmune disorders, and Alzheimer's.[23]

Low blood sugar levels drive many people to eat unhealthy foods. That's why it's important to focus first on trying to heal the body. Most people, including many doctors, don't consider weight loss, and more generally our body and our health, from the integrated, whole-person-first clinical perspective that we've been discussing.

Yet doing so would pay healthy dividends!

We first need to focus on what is essential and on what will help our body to better self-regulate. Along the way, that includes helping to normalize weight. When your body loses its ability to self-regulate, to heal, and to maintain good function, you can end up engaging in eating behaviors that you know aren't good for you but that you find hard to stop.

Those who have low blood sugar levels can reduce this issue by eating more frequently and eating the right types of foods. Many with this type of problem like to skip breakfast, knowing that they probably will be munching on junk food later that day.

They shouldn't skip breakfast because their blood sugar levels may be too low in the morning. That may lead them to feel weak or have cravings for high-calorie foods later.

For people who suffer from low blood sugar, it's important to have an adequate amount of protein with each meal. Maintaining a steady level of protein throughout the day can keep blood sugar levels more balanced and can affect the appetite center of the brain so that one feels less hungry. One of the benefits of protein is that it activates a type of brain receptor that triggers satiety, a satisfied feeling of being full.

Another way to help heal this condition is to eat snacks between meals with good protein content and complex carbohydrates. Nonstarchy vegetables are usually a good choice. If you have had difficulty maintaining stable blood sugar levels, this will help your body to normalize them.

Many people with this type of issue eat the way they do because their body feels weak, so they run to the things that will instantly put sugar in the blood for the body to use—refined carbohydrates. These types of carbs raise the level of glucose, or sugar, in your blood more quickly than table sugar, believe it or not.

Doing this also temporarily raises the level of the neurotransmitters serotonin, which I mentioned earlier helps to make people feel calmer, and dopamine, which also alters your mood. As a result, a lot of people not just report having more energy but also admit that they feel better emotionally after eating those types of foods.

There is catch, however. Eating a lot of junk food creates a temporary spike in your blood sugar level, which then drops quickly because your insulin level rises sharply. Chronic higher-than-normal insulin levels increase inflammation and can lead to increased plaque in your blood vessels. High insulin levels are also associated with greater incidence of certain cancers and can stimulate the liver to produce fatty substances that go into the bloodstream.[24]

On a long-term basis, they can disrupt the creation of feel-good neurotransmitters in your brain, making you want to snack on junk food more often.

Once again, we see a connection that creates a vicious cycle. On top of that, high insulin levels also stimulate fat storage.[25,26]

So a good way to help control fat levels in your blood is to normalize your insulin levels.

High insulin levels also have an effect on active thyroid hormones, which we discussed earlier. If your liver becomes resistant to insulin, it can no longer efficiently convert the inactive hormone created in your thyroid to the active type that your cells respond to.

It's another example of how a lab test could show that the thyroid is producing a normal level of hormones when the body could be expressing thyroid insufficiency symptoms, such as the ones previously mentioned: depression, weight gain, digestive issues, hair loss, and others.

Remember, high levels of the stress hormone cortisol can also do that to you. People can experience a number of other negative effects due to chronic high insulin levels, but what is of immediate importance for the sake of our discussion on weight is that chronic high insulin levels decrease your body's ability to burn fat.

Sugar and insulin levels should rise and fall within a healthy functional range, depending on whether you are in a fasting stage or have recently eaten.

Some of our favorite restaurants can help or hurt our body's ability to handle sugar levels, depending what we order from the menu.

With visions of fried rice and fortune cookies, let's use Chinese food as an example, as well as discuss topics that can help you understand and handle the dynamics of stress and its connection to being overweight.

What You Can Do Now

- Help reduce your pain by lowering inflammation. Help reduce inflammation by decreasing excess fat tissue, which produces inflammatory compounds.
- If you are tired during the day, yet you wake up often in the middle of the night without the need to uri-

nate, check with your doctor to see if you have low cortisol levels. If you get irritated before meals, feel a lot better after meals, and crave sweets in between, you may be suffering from low blood sugar. Low cortisol levels may be the cause.

- If you typically feel weak between meals and have urges to snack on sugary or refined carbs before you eat again, consider high-protein snacks instead. They help to stabilize your blood sugar levels.

- Find that you overeat often? A lot of my patients report that after they feel healthier and start to lose weight, they lose their urges to overeat. Be patient with your body in the beginning . . . and also your brain, as it begins to modify its responses to the volume of foods eaten.

- The types of bacteria found in our gut are associated with either weight loss or obesity. Generally speaking, Bacteroidetes concentrations were lower in obese people,[27] while Firmicutes concentrations were higher. Manipulating the composition of your gut flora through probiotics and prebiotics is helpful in losing weight.[28,29,30,31,32]

- Emotionally slouched? Remember that sitting upright decreases cortisol levels, boosts testosterone levels, and makes it easier to change your mood. Fake it (for just two minutes) until you make it!

[21]

Your Hormones and Stress

HISTORICALLY, CHINESE RESTAURANTS in the United States have served foods loaded with refined carbohydrates and starches, such as noodles, but with little protein. These carbs and starches bring up your blood sugar level quickly, and your body reacts by releasing a lot of insulin, which drives your blood sugar level down.

The low blood sugar can trigger hunger pangs. If you eat this type of food, or other foods that are similar, consider eating adequate amounts of protein with the meal to help stabilize your blood sugar levels.

Since we're on the topic of Chinese food, the Buddha said that on life's journey, faith is nourishment. In the Mandarin language, the verbs for "eat food" and "take medicine" are written the same way.

Many people's bodies are under a lot of physical, mental, emotional, or other types of stress. Maybe your body isn't healthy. An unhealthy body tends to lead to unhealthy choices, including mental and emotional ones, which in turn drive this negative loop.

But you can change that!

Let's explore what we can learn from how our bodies respond to stress and how it has an effect on what we end up eating. We discussed how food can alter how your brain works and how you feel, that it is not just about feeling full or taking in energy. Now let's focus a little more deeply on stress. Let's define it and discuss how it affects us. This is important because it ties in with what I have been emphasizing regarding multiple causes associated with chronic conditions and illnesses.

People can respond to the same type of environmental input, whether emotional, mental, or physical, in different ways. Stress isn't necessarily bad. It's how you respond to it that determines its effect on your body.

In the 1930s, a Canadian doctor by the name of Hans Selye defined stress in terms of its effect on the body. Good stress, which you could handle well and benefit from, he called "eustress." Stress that was not handled well and was harmful to the body he termed "distress."[1,2,3,4]

In his laboratory experiments, the common changes he found in the body as a result of long-term distress included an increase in stomach ulcers; a reduction in the size of lymph tissue, which is part of your immune system; and an enlargement of the adrenal glands, which we mentioned also create stress-related hormones, such as cortisol and catecholamines.[5,6,7,8,9,10,11]

However, as Selye noted, it's how you respond to stress that determines whether it will be beneficial or harmful. In other words, it's usually how you emotionally and mentally react to a situation that makes a difference. That difference can make changes in your body, for better or for worse.

Changing your viewpoints, how you see things, makes a tangible difference in your health.

Research shows that people who feel more connected to others get sick less often and those who have a happy marriage have fewer heart issues, regardless of other variables. Even just looking at the glass as half-full can make a clinical difference. People who are optimistic have a significantly lower risk of death.[12,13,14,15,16]

The earnest clinician takes into account all aspects of a person's experiences, not just laboratory or imaging findings or the results of a physical examination. Sometimes, listening has a greater therapeutic benefit than prescribing. There are times when a friendly ear can heal more than a good prescription.

In an earlier chapter, we discussed some tools that can help you cope better with stress. We will go over more of them later.

Stress and Hormones

Before we leave this topic, I'd like to touch on one more aspect of high cortisol levels and their connection to female hormones.

Chronic high cortisol levels, produced by stress, create a resistance in the body to practically all other hormones, including thyroid hormones and female hormones. These include progesterone and the three main types of estrogens.

There are receptors in cells of the brain that respond to estrogen. It's well-known that hot flashes, for example, can be a symptom of estrogen deficiency.[17,18]

Cellular receptors that respond to estrogen can be affected by chronic high levels of cortisol, the chronic-stress hormone. Women with higher levels of cortisol during the transitional stage of menopause have more severe hot flashes than those with lower levels of cortisol, despite having the same estrogen levels.[19]

Guess what could happen to someone you know in that phase of her life whose blood tests showed normal levels of estrogen but who had experienced chronic stress, which kept her cortisol levels high for too long?

Her brain would be less responsive to her estrogen levels because the chronically high cortisol levels would affect her receptors for estrogen. So she could start having hot flashes, but the blood work could show normal estrogen levels.

If she had hot flashes as a result of this and went to a doctor who only gave her estrogen supplementation without looking for the underlying causes of her hot flashes, she could end up with medicine that was addressing an effect rather than correcting a cause.

Unequal Supplements

Every healthy garden needs good soil, and good soil needs water, worms, and the right amount of micronutrients to feed the garden's plants and help them to grow. Good soil also makes a difference in our health—many of the organisms living in the roots of plants we eat have at least one important function that we know of.

Researchers found that these microorganisms help transform inorganic minerals into organic minerals so that we can more easily assimilate them into our bodies. That's why inorganic minerals found in many supplements are often not helpful. Healthy, living soil is important for our health.

Unfortunately, our soil today doesn't contain the variety and amount of minerals and other nutrients that were present in the soil of our forefathers.[20,21,22]

As helpful as medicine can be at times for certain conditions, we still need our body, like a garden, to work in a balanced, nutrient-rich, and harmonious way to benefit best from whatever therapeutic approach is used, from organic carrots to cardiac surgery.

Regarding supplements, there are times when your body might respond best to higher dosages of vitamins and minerals that are found in our foods. My experience has been that supplements based on foods, and not synthetically created in a laboratory, however, usually give us the best chance for long-term healing.

Not all vitamins are created the same. As with nature, supplementing is more complex than just dosage. In terms of how your body absorbs and benefits from them, think of most vitamins as you would a family member.

Your family is there to support you, right? The nutritional equivalent of that support in the body is known as *cofactors,* which help many vitamins, minerals, and other nutrients to work better.

Many supplements include nutritional products consisting of isolated, synthetic vitamins that are missing these essential cofactors. Many prescriptions, over-the-counter products, online vitamins, and clinician-sold supplements might contain high doses of synthetic vitamins, which are often derived from coal tar, petroleum, and genetically modified corn syrup.

There are about five pharmaceutical corporations in the United States that make most of these synthetic vitamins, selling them to vitamin and nutritional supply companies. But you won't read "synthetic" on the bottle.

Our food contains thousands of important micronutrients. These cofactors, or helpers, are found in the whole foods that you eat, which leads to another important point: nature knows more than we do. For example, there are over 25,000 active compounds created naturally in plants, termed *phytochemicals,* which are important to your health and healing.

Synthetic or artificial vitamins often lack essential cofactors, which complete and balance the whole nutrient complex. These include a number of phytochemicals. Synthetic vitamins can create nutritional deficiencies because of these missing cofactors and nutrients. Many of these necessary nutrients, found in nature, have not yet been discovered.

As we become more aware of how nature works, scientists have become more aware of the benefits of and the need for biodiversity globally. Nature created a multiplicity whose abundance is recognized more and more as essential for the health of our planet.

Our body is part of nature. Why not take that same approach with our food and our supplements?

You can't create these biologically active compounds in a lab and put them in a supplement bottle. A vegetable has many hundreds of them. That's why it's best to eat foods in their natural state and then supplement with food-based products as necessary. Resort to laboratory-created supplements only if really needed. Since we know so little of all that nature has to offer us, why not, paradoxically, help our bodies to heal through the wisdom of ignorance?

That is, eat foods in their whole state, because that is how nature created them. Assume that there are proportions and unknown ingredients whose sum is greater than the parts. That helps us move beyond what we can see through the limitations of our microscopes and lab analyses.

This subject often leads people to ask about organic foods, which are usually more expensive. One frequently asked question is whether organic foods have more nutritional value. There's been a lot of debate about this in the media. A lot of people think that organic foods have about the same amount of minerals and nutrition as conventionally grown crops.

The research is not definitive in terms of what are known as the usual macro minerals, such as calcium, potassium, and magnesium. We do see a lot of variation when these macronutrient numbers are compared, depending on the study involved.

Nutritional testing is growing more sophisticated, however. It will always have limits, yet it's revealing more information about smaller but important biologically active compounds in foods.

One class of these compounds—mentioned previously, is known as *phytochemicals.* There are thousands of them, with new ones being discovered every month. You don't see them listed on most vitamin bottles.

Metabolomics is the study of the chemical effects of these small molecules. Research that uses metabolomic approaches highlights the advantages that organic foods seem to offer. This research has demonstrated on a consistent basis that many organic foods have a greater quantity of many of these biologically active compounds, the phytochemicals. These include antioxidants and cancer-fighting agents.[23,24,25,26]

Organically fed chicken showed stronger immune responses than conventionally fed ones, according to one study. Selenium is a mineral that our bodies need for cellular function; sows that were fed from organic selenium sources had piglets that had higher levels of it than those fed from inorganic sources, and the sows retained more of it in their tissues.[27]

Pesticides

There are also times when commonly used pesticides in conventionally grown foods can interfere with a plant's mineral absorption and affect its chlorophyll content.[28,29,30,31,32,33]

So there is a lot to be said for looking more closely at the benefits of organic foods, beyond the pesticides and genetic manipulation issues usually associated with conventional foods.[34,35,36,37,38]

To illustrate the effect that pesticides have on children, here's an example. If children switch to organic foods, certain organophosphorus pesticides commonly used in conventional agriculture drop to undetectable levels in their urine in five days. When they start eating conventional foods, the pesticide levels in their urine jump right back up again.[39]

Think about it: in less than a week your kids can go from showing traces of pesticide in their urine to undetectable levels, simply by eating organic food.

It's important, for adults as well as children, because pesticide exposure can change the way your immune system works. Most people have detectable exposure to pesticides, which can depress the body's immune responses, as well as affect fertility.[40,41,42,43,44,45]

Children, moreover, are more biologically vulnerable to the effects of pesticides than adults. When you look into the eyes of a young child, keep in mind that the rest of her organs, where pesticides have stronger metabolic effects, are proportionally larger than those of an adult and are still developing, which creates a window of vulnerability.

Young children drink more water and eat more food per pound than do adults; a six-month-old drinks seven times more water for his weight than an adult. Their immature bodies also have more difficulty detoxifying pesticides than adults. Injury to brain cells and disruptions in the development of their organs and glands from pesticides have been shown to cause permanent, irreversible damage.[46]

In rural Minnesota, children of parents who applied pesticides in farms were found to have significantly higher rates of birth defects.[47] Research has shown that children exposed to weed killers have a higher incidence of attention deficit disorders, hyperactivity, and asthma.[48,49]

Beyond the issue of health food sources, we need to keep in mind that there is more to food than simply nutrition. Nutrition serves as the building blocks for our cells and tissues. But food also has another important purpose: cellular information.

Herbs That Help

Beyond the carbs, fats, proteins, minerals, and vitamins that food provides, which are what we generally call nutrition, food also provides natural chemicals that stimulate receptors in many cells of our body. In doing so, they help the cells respond in ways that are healthy for us.

Take herbs, for instance. For thousands of years, they have been used to help heal our wounds and illnesses. Their primary beneficial effect isn't in the carbs or protein, or even in the minerals that they contain. It's in the particular makeup of these active biological chemicals, these phytochemicals, as well as other ingredients that science has not yet discovered, which serve as a call to action for the cells of our body to respond to their health challenges, to help us heal.

Recently, Western medicine has focused more on a healing concept that has been around for thousands of years. The modern name for it is *immunotherapy*. Basically, it's about finding ways to help the immune system fight many diseases, including cancer.

However, herbs have been used for this purpose throughout history. Modern research is now finally documenting the benefits of this age-old approach. This is another example of how connecting with the healing wisdom of older traditions is helpful. In medieval England, even the most modest of Tudor homes had an herbal garden for healing, with herbal remedies passed down from family to family. Some countries, such as China, with a long history of using herbs for healing, are leading scientific research in this area.[50,51,52,53,54]

These immune-system helpers are not just found in herbs. Foods that we eat every day have them as well. But it seems that organic food has the edge over conventionally grown food in providing more of these active biological compounds.[55,56,57,58,59,60,61,62,63,64,65,66,67,68,69]

Besides their more commonly known benefits regarding the absence of pesticides, toxins, and genetic modifications, organic foods shine at providing these biological health and healing agents.

In the next chapter, we are going to go deeper into the topic of helping you to lose weight. One of the main themes of this book is to look at things differently to get different results, to see health from an expanded point of view. In that vein, consider this: if sick dogs have taught us something about our eating habits, what do you think a mirror could teach us about weight loss?

What You Can Do Now

- If you want to explore how your viewpoints are affecting your stress levels and overall health, one consideration is online cognitive behavioral therapy. Harvard Medical School has a website with more information, which can be found at harvard.edu.
- One of the hormones released by chronic stress, cortisol, negatively affects practically all of your body systems. Find ways to release the stress to lower effects of this hormone. Some have been outlined in a previous chapter.
- Some see the glass half full; others see the glass half empty . . . be grateful that you have something in

your glass at all! Gratitude for what you do have paves the inner road to recovery.

- If you are a loner or feel isolated, join a community group that you would feel comfortable with. You will get sick less often.

- Whole-food supplements contain thousands of biologically active components not found in chemically created supplements. Use whole-food supplements as a daily foundation, and add specific products when needed.

- It's often what you don't see or feel that has long-term destructive effects on your health and that of your children, such as exposure to pesticides, either in the food you serve them or outside. Buying organic foods, at least while your children are young and especially vulnerable, decreases their risk of having brain and body health issues down the road.

[22]

Mirror, Mirror

I MENTIONED THAT different body types seem to do better with different types of weight-loss plans. It seems that foods that help one person lose weight might not be as helpful for someone with a different body type.[1,2]

This is where the mirror metaphor comes in. If you want to change an image that you don't like when you look into a mirror, would it make sense to try to change the mirror?

Of course not! The mirror is just a reflection of whatever is in front of it. It's the same thing with being overweight. The shape of your body is really just a reflection, a mirror, of what is taking place inside of you. It's typically the long-term consequence of the relationship between body functions, including metabolism, and your historical interaction with food.

To change the mirror's reflection, its image, it's best to begin changing the internal processes within your body that have led to the shape that your mirror shows.

The foundation of any clinical approach to help you lose weight should include determining which other body functions need to be helped, because often those are the root causes of being overweight, which is usually just an expression, a consequence.

Some people have a genetic predisposition to obesity, but generally speaking, research has not found that these genes have a large influence on weight when compared with lifestyle decisions. And for those who do have these genes, the studies show that heredity is not destiny.

As usual in the field of science, there is some research as well, however, that shows differently. In this case, a study has been published showing, for the first time, a genetic link between the way your body handles digestion of carbs and obesity.

A study that was published in 2014 pointed to a strong genetic connection between obesity and gene variance. The research involved more than 6,000 subjects. They looked at obese people and those with certain structural genetic variations of the type known as copy number variations, or CNVs, which I previously mentioned also have an effect on Crohn's as well as a number of other diseases.

CNVs, as I noted, are different than the single nucleotide polymorphisms, or SNPs, that are advertised for testing in the media. CNVs are structural genetic changes and are more widespread than SNPs.

The results demonstrate that subjects with lower copy numbers of the gene for salivary amylase, which is an enzyme in your saliva that helps to digest starch, had an eight-times-greater risk for obesity as those with the highest copy numbers. People in countries where more starches are eaten, such as Asia, tend to have a higher number of copies of this gene, and typically have lower body fat.[3]

We need to focus on processes and functions that aren't working well in the body, and help to heal dysfunctional processes that contribute to weight gain. Lifestyle habits also need to be taken into consideration.

Body-Weight Set Points

On the subject of persistent obesity and genetics, what about those who seem to be doing everything right and still have more difficulty losing weight than others? Let's spend some time going over an interesting theory that may help to account for this: the body-weight set point theory.

Basically, this theory proposes that our body functions to keep us at a certain weight.[4,5,6] There are other theories that also revolve around this sticky-weight concept, such as the settling points theory, the general intake theory, and the dual intervention point model,[7] but for the purposes of this discussion we will put our attention on the body-weight set point theory.

You can think of it as a thermostat for your weight scale. Your hormones, neurotransmitters, rate of energy expenditure, and tissues work to defend a stable weight range. Genetic influence also matters. If you eat more than usual, your body will metabolize the energy from the fat more quickly to help to move you back to your regular weight. If you eat less than usual, such as losing weight through a diet, according to this theory, your body will slow down how quickly it uses its energy reserves so that your weight goes back up![8,9,10]

Unfortunately, research along the lines of this model shows something that you have already experienced: your body will put weight back on more quickly than it loses it. People with a high body-weight set point will weigh more, and have more difficulty keeping the weight off, while those with a lower set point weigh less, and will find it easier to move back to the lower weight after gaining weight over time due to overeating.[11]

Other research points to the effects of yo-yo dieting on your metabolism, your fat-burning rate. Continuing to start and stop diet plans can make it twice as hard to lose the weight, and three times as easy to gain weight.[12] I mentioned before that your thyroid hormones, which help to control your metabolism, don't work as effectively when you go on severe diets.[13,14,15] This reduction in how your thyroid hormones work inside your cells is not usually picked up by laboratory testing.[16,17,18]

Obese people who are exposed to certain types of pesticides and pollutants may have increased weight set points. These can be due to the results of the effects of these chemicals on enzymes and metabolic function.[19]

Have you noticed how often people who stop smoking gain weight, and vice versa? It turns out that nicotine lowers the weight set point. The increased set point upon withdrawal of use is one reason why there is often a weight increase.[20]

If you have a high body-weight set point, assuming that this theory holds true, what do you do? It may be more difficult for you to lose and keep the weight off past a certain point.

If it is true, however, there is hope. You can still lose the weight and keep it off. Following the suggestions in this book would be more important for you than ever. A steady approach, and patience, will yield rewards.

Some of the things that you can do to help to bring down your set point include making sure that your diet choices do not lead to insulin resistance, or chronic high insulin levels. Lowering your insulin levels, along with an increase in another blood-sugar-regulating hormone, known as glucagon, may lower your set point level.[21]

Another way that you can help to lower your body-weight set point is to have stable blood sugar levels. Even mild levels of low blood sugar have been shown to be linked with subsequent weight gain—as well as a greater risk of developing diabetes.[22]

There's more you can do to help yourself to lower your body-weight set point. Exercise helps.[23] Even the way that genes associated with obesity express themselves can change. It's known as epigenetics. Gene function can change through lifestyle modifications.

Other ways to help reset your body-weight set point involve eating more protein. In a study that involved overweight and obese Canadian women, those who ate a high-protein diet, consisting of 1 gram of protein for every gram of carbohydrate consumed, had higher resting metabolic rates at the end of the study period. When compared with a control group eating a conventional diet, where three grams of carbohydrates were consumed for every gram of protein, the 1:1 carb/protein group also had decreased amounts of cholesterol.

The researchers concluded that a high-protein diet, even without doing exercise, was actually better in promoting weight loss than a low-fat, high-carbohydrate diet that included exercise![24]

The takeaway from that study, and others, is that a high-protein diet, combined with exercise, gives the greatest benefit.[25,26] Other research also points to the benefits of strength training to help to lower your body-weight set point.[27] On the other hand, high-fat diets can lead to higher body-weight set points.[28]

It's not just the number of calories; it's the type that also matters. Eating higher levels of quality protein, lowering fat intake levels below those found in the usual American diet, eating low-glycemic-load veggies (see chapter 27), and doing exercise will help you to shift your body-weight set point.

More help: lower the levels of inflammation in your body, keeping in mind that some foods are inflammatory to many people, and that others may have inflammatory reactions to some foods universally deemed as healthy.

Chronic inflammation sets off a pattern of anti-inflammatory responses in your body, including high levels of cortisol, which I mentioned also works as an anti-inflammatory hormone in your body. Lowering cortisol levels can help to lower your body-weight set point.[29]

On a similar note, you may remember that we spoke of cortisol as the body's main chronic stress hormone. Therefore, lifestyle changes and body-mind, as well as mind-body, approaches that help you to lower your stress levels may also be helpful (see chapter 16). A number of them are highlighted throughout this book.

Losing Fat or Muscle?

If you are on the right clinical program, losing weight does not necessarily mean that you lost a lot of fat. Many people who go on crash weight-loss programs end up losing a lot of muscle. Muscle weighs more than fat, and we want to maintain or even increase the amount of muscle in our body while losing the fat. Fat takes up much more space in the body but does not weigh as much as muscle, since muscle is approximately 20 percent denser.[30,31,32]

This is why many of us would be better off putting more attention on our body shape than on the bathroom scale. I'm more interested when patients tell me that they are seeing the inches come off their waist and hips, and that they are able to wear smaller dress or pant sizes, even though the scale does not show as big a weight loss as they would have expected.

Muscle burns a lot of calories throughout the day and night as well, even if you're not exercising, so having good muscle tone is important for continued weight loss. I remember a patient who gained a pound after a few weeks of dieting and exercise, which included weight-lifting. She was happy that her waist had reduced in size during that time. She gained muscle and lost fat!

If a person gains around four pounds of muscle, then he or she can lose around 20 pounds in the next four years just through the extra calories those extra muscles will use, without doing anything different. With just a one-time addition of just four pounds of additional muscle, the caloric equivalent of five pounds is burned off, year after year.[33,34]

Studies show a relationship between illnesses, decreased muscle mass, and increased fat percentage in adults. Having more muscle mass can lower sugar levels in the blood and reduce insulin resistance.[35,36,37,38,39,40]

Unfortunately, waistlines are expanding in the United States; they have grown over an inch in the past decade or so. Fat around the waist is the worst type to have, as we will discuss later. However, research has shown that the average body mass index measurement has not changed. And for that to happen while body fat has increased, the amount of muscle mass has decreased.[41]

I stress losing fat instead of simply looking at the scale, although you will see that you will weigh less as well. Losing weight naturally, and in a way that makes it easy to keep off, has a much better chance of taking place in a healthier body, where supporting systems are working the way they should.

And that's how the image in the mirror changes!

Diet and exercise alone are usually not enough for most people to make permanent changes in their weight. Not because they aren't worthwhile: in fact, they should be followed. Rather, most people who try only a diet and exercise program gain the weight back in a matter of months. We talked about international research showing that no nation from the 188 studied has seen a decline in obesity rates in the past 33 years.

So what's going on?

What's happening is that our bodies are not ready to sustain losing weight for long enough periods of time. I mentioned that research shows that up to 80 percent of those who lose weight gain it back within 12 months. A number of them end up weighing more.[42,43,44]

Most people attribute a failed diet to a lack of discipline. They grit their teeth and promise to try again . . . and again, and again.

For many, learning about the connections between fluctuations in hormones such as cortisol, blood sugar levels, and other elements that we will discuss later can help them to understand how their body can be helped by putting attention on all the systems that help one to heal.

While discipline and desire play an important and needed role in sustained weight loss, along with exercise and proper eating, for many people there is much more to it.

To stress this point, sometimes I offer patients—for those who don't have body challenges that are a contraindication—what I call the hundred-dollar breath challenge. I tell them that if they can hold their breath for two minutes, I will give them a hundred-dollar bill.

A number have tried. Afterward, many have asked me, breathlessly, what this challenge had to do with weight loss. I tell them that you can have all the enthusiasm and discipline in the world, but if your body isn't prepared for it, you are not going to meet the goal, whether it is holding your breath long enough or staying on a sustained weight-loss program.

What's the weight-loss equivalent of the hundred-dollar breath test in your body?

What You Can Do Now

- Focus on changing how the inside of your body works first in order to make the weight come off easier and longer. If despite endless diet and exercise plans over the years, the shape in the mirror hasn't changed, ask yourself what else in your mind-body functions needs to undergo changes.
- If you think that you may have a high body-weight set point, making it harder to keep the weight off, be kind and patient with your body. Know that your body will not be as forgiving as others if you fall off the proverbial weight-loss wagon. Exercise, make

sure that you eat higher than usual levels of good-quality protein, lower the usual fat intake, and eat nonstarchy veggies to give you the upper hand. Hang in there—eventually you'll make it!

- Lose fat and not muscle by exercising and realizing that nice and steady is the best way to lose it. Concentrate on losing the fat stores around your waist and hips, and keeping the muscle.
- Lose volume, not density!

[23]

Secrets to Weight Loss?

MOST PEOPLE, EVEN if healthy, would never be able to hold their breath for two minutes unless they had specialized training, like big-wave surfers or deep-sea divers. Most of my patients who have tried it don't last 60 seconds.

Just because you want something badly, whether holding your breath for a while or losing weight, it doesn't mean that your body is ready to do it. There are things your body needs to be doing to lose weight and to keep the weight off. You need to be able to lose weight without hunger, energy loss, or feeling bad.

One thing you need to focus on when losing weight is the importance of losing fat, not muscle. Certain diet programs promise weight loss, but they don't specify where the weight comes from. A lot of them end up costing you muscle mass, which you don't want to lose. A number of these weight-loss programs can work against your best interests.

If you reduce your daily caloric intake too much, for instance, your body's resting metabolic rate can reset itself so that it burns calories more slowly.[1] Your body is using the calories that you eat more efficiently, which will make it harder to lose weight. If that happens, it means that while you are resting, your body can be up to 20 percent more efficient at not using up calories.[2] That's important because most of the calories your body burns in a day are burned when you're not doing much.

On the other hand, and this goes to the point earlier in this book about contradictions in science, I also read studies praising the effects of intermittent fasting for health and weight loss. At the end of the day, you need to see what works for you, for your body, which is unique.

Burning Calories

Let's talk about your body and calories.

There are three ways in which your body burns calories in a day, also known as *total daily energy expenditure*.

1. The first is through the resting metabolic rate. This is what your body maintains throughout the day to keep its body temperature working well and to regulate your organ systems. We talked about the thyroid gland and its importance in helping to regulate this. The resting metabolic rate accounts for most of your calories burned—around 65 percent of them.[3]

2. The second way that your body burns energy is through the thermal effect of physical activity, including exercise. It accounts for up to 25 percent of your total calories burned in a day, depending on how active you are.[4] How can you increase the number of calories you burn when you are not able to exercise? There are things you can do to help yourself. Done as a daily habit, they can make a difference. It can be as simple as taking the stairs instead of the elevator or escalator, or parking your car a little farther away from the office than usual, or walking a bit quicker than normal. You could also stand up at work more instead of always sitting. It's the frequency of these little things, done throughout the day, that's important. Do them day in and day out. Turn them into little daily habits that over time will make a big weight difference.
3. The third way in which we burn calories involves the energy it takes to digest and process the food we eat. That can be as much as 10 percent of your total daily energy expenditure.[5,6] The typical man burns the equivalent of two pounds a month just using energy to handle all aspects of food digestion.[7,8]

Yes, you burn calories by eating!

In fact, a number of people with insulin resistance get tired after meals, especially heavy meals, because on the one hand they are using up energy to digest the food, but on the other hand the cells of the body resist accepting sugar, or glucose, to use as a fuel. They feel tired as a result, wanting to take a nap after eating.

A lot of these people like to eat something sweet after a meal because it provides a quick (but short) burst of energy. Another reason why people with insulin resistance, and others, can feel sleepy after meals is because their levels of the neurotransmitters GABA and serotonin temporarily increase.

Speaking of burning calories, did you know that you have approximately six pounds of body weight that burns almost 40 percent of all your calories in one day, and that it's not muscle?

Remember that we said your liver weighs around three pounds? Your brain weighs roughly the same. Both of them combined account for between 35 and 40 percent of your daily energy expenditure.[9] The brain and the liver are metabolically active. They are busy calorie-burning organs!

We've been talking about losing weight by burning fat in the usual sense, but think about these questions for a moment: Do you really "burn it off" or "melt the fat"? Does fat convert to muscle?

The answer to these questions is no!

Most of the weight loss that you experience is breathed out as carbon dioxide, believe it or not.[10]

Let's suppose that you recently lost 10 pounds. To do that, over that period of time you exhaled the equivalent of approximately eight pounds by breathing out carbon dioxide. The other pound or so was lost through the release of water in breath and bodily fluids. For those who think they see a shortcut here, hyperventilation will not help you to lose weight, and it might leave you feeling dizzy or worse.[11]

Since your brain is burning so many calories (your fat-burning friend!), you can see why having low blood sugar is not going to work well if you want to have a brain that feels alert. Blood sugar issues can leave you feeling tired and lightheaded, and can make it hard to concentrate.

Muscle Matters

Now that you know the resting metabolic rate is what burns up most of your calories in a day, you should be able to see why you want to keep good muscle tone as you lose weight. I mentioned before how a few pounds of extra muscle can lead to pounds of weight loss year after year, everything else being equal.

As I said in the previous chapter, adding just four pounds of muscle can mean losing five pounds a year, year after year, assuming nothing else has changed, simply because of the extra energy burned by the additional muscle.

That amounts to the equivalent of 50 pounds over a space of 10 years. However, there is a flip side to this—and it's not good news.

It's not easy to gain muscle, but it is easy to lose it. People go on extreme, energy-restrictive diet plans to lose a lot of pounds in a month. The average person doing moderate daily exercise typically loses around four pounds of body fat per month. That's it—it's not much. Bear in mind that I'm talking about fat, not weight. The rest is mostly water and muscle.[12,13,14,15,16,17,18,19]

We don't want to lose muscle. If having more muscle helps us to lose weight over the long term, then losing muscle while dieting will make it more difficult to keep the weight off later.[20,21] As you might have experienced, or know of others who have had the experience, the weight will usually pack back on, and then some. It takes patience.

A Little Exercise That Goes a Long Way

When someone is attempting to lose weight, it is important that he or she exercise, preferably doing resistance training, which means working with weights or against resistance. This helps to spare muscle loss during a diet program. Fat can still be lost with low-protein diets, but diets that are higher in protein compared with a standard diet help retain more muscle mass.[22]

The good news is that there is a way to spend a lot less time exercising and yet lose more weight and fat.

I've already suggested resistance or weight training. If you combine this with moderate-intensity aerobics, you'll have one of the best combinations possible to lose weight. These exercises will decrease weight and belly fat more than any other specific exercise approach, including aerobics alone.[23,24,25]

If you want to focus on doing a fair amount of moderate exercise, you have to exercise for only 30 minutes a day, five days a week. Remember: moderate exercise. Don't kill yourself. Research has shown that doing high-intensity exercises for a long time will not help you lose more weight.

There is some interesting research, however, that recommends doing high-intensity exercises for short spurts of 30 seconds or so, followed by a minute of rest, then another all-out spurt for 30 seconds, then going easy for a minute, then repeating. A few minutes of this type of short-spurt exercise is enough for a great workout. Some research points to waiting longer, three to four minutes, before doing another full-intensity 30-second spurt, as the extra recuperation time can help to increase your peak heart rate the second time.

This type of exercise has shown to be as effective as doing much longer low- or moderate-intensity exercise.[26,27] This type of interval training helps your cardiovascular system, improves muscle tone, helps you to lose weight, and helps trigger beneficial brain changes too. You can do it on a treadmill, on a stationary bike, or running upstairs and using the rest time to slowly walk down. The important thing is to do maximal efforts with the large muscle groups of your body. Check with your trainer and get medical clearance if you need to. You can get your exercise done in four high-intensity minutes a day, with rests in between!

For those with insulin resistance or diabetes, these types of short, maximum-intensity exercises also have the benefits of helping the receptors in the cells of the body to accept insulin more easily and of decreasing blood sugar levels.[28,29] You can do most of these exercises at home, meaning that you don't have to stay in those hour-long classes.

One of the many fringe benefits to exercise is that your body usually burns around 100 calories after you finish a session of moderate-intensity exercise. The more intense the exercise, the more fat is burned after the exercise is finished. This is known as the *afterburn effect,* or excess post-exercise oxygen consumption. It does not sound like much, but 100 calories a day adds up to 12 pounds a year of fat loss as a side effect of doing daily exercise. That's on top of the calories that you burned while exercising!

Get it done, and lose more fat in half the time or less![30,31] I noted that exercise also helps increase brain function, especially high-intensity exercise. Yet, even for highly active people, physical training isn't enough to cause a big change in the percentage of fat in your body unless it's accompanied by a sound nutritional plan.[33,33,34] If you don't exercise and eat enough protein, it can lead to greater muscle loss during a weight-loss program.[35,36,37,38]

Preparing to Lose Weight More Easily

Eating appropriately and working out are important. However, the body needs to be as healthy as possible to support the results of diet and exercise to lose weight—and, optimally, to lose fat, not muscle.

Beyond eating healthy and in moderation, as well as exercising when the body is ready, most people need to start by focusing on a number of body dynamics, important connections that make the difference to you to lose weight with more ease.

One is the need to make sure that there are no interferences in the master system—the nervous system—of the body, which helps the organs and tissues to communicate well with the brain. It is an important aspect of good health and vitality.

Research shows that, for many, obesity is associated with increased activity of the stress response—this is the fight-or-flight-response part of our nervous system, the sympathetic nervous system.[39,40,41,42,43,44,45,46,47,48,49,50,51,52,53,54,55]

Studies have shown that modulating the primary digestive nerve, called the *vagus* nerve, has led to decreased weight and fat levels.[56,57] The U.S. Food and Drug Administration has approved a device that blocks the nerve to control hunger and fullness.[58]

Chiropractic care affects how the nervous system works. It has a modulating effect on the nervous system and on the immune system. I am not suggesting that this type of care is an instrument for weight loss. Rather, it can be a part, when necessary, of a number of good approaches to better health, which is needed for a successful return to normal weight.

It's important to decrease chronic inflammatory processes in the body, since inflammation can make it harder to lose weight.

Inflammation does have an effect on weight loss. Acute inflammatory reactions in your body are normal and helpful. Chronic inflammation, however, is harmful for a number of reasons. As it relates to weight control, chronic inflammation affects the brain center that is responsible for feeling full and satisfied when you are eating. You may remember that we discussed that eating protein helps us to feel full and satisfied quicker.

Elevated levels of cortisol also increase insulin, helping to stop the breakdown of fat. Chronic inflammation, which many people have even if they don't feel pain, can have a negative impact on a number of body functions. That makes it much harder to lose weight.

You might remember when I mentioned earlier that the arcuate nucleus of the hypothalamus in your brain is the main hunger center. Chronic inflammation increases cortisol levels because cortisol is an anti-inflammatory, and it's also released by the body in response to continued stress, whether physical or emotional stress.

Chronic high cortisol levels can affect your appetite, making it harder to eat less.

When you eat, hormones are released from your fat cells that go to this part of your brain and make you feel full and satisfied. However, chronic elevated cortisol levels increase the levels of one of these hormones released by your fat cells, called leptin, to the point that the body develops leptin resistance, making it harder for the appetite center to recognize that it is full. As a result, you end up eating more.[59,60]

You can help your body to lose weight by supporting its proper adrenal gland function, reducing cortisol levels, improving digestion, and making sure that your liver and detoxifying systems, such as your kidneys, work well.

However, for many patients, detoxifying is not the first step. They simply aren't ready for that. Organs, glands, and systems need to be healthy to handle the extra toxin-load release by the tissues during a detoxifying program. Your body's drainage systems—in effect, your garbage pickup and disposal systems, such as your lymphatic, intestinal, liver, and kidney functions, along with your lungs, and even your skin—need to be working well.

Detoxifying is part of what the body goes through as you lose weight. People whose body is not healthy enough to easily undergo detoxification can find weight loss a challenge.

Later you'll see why key organs have to work well to help you lose weight more easily. It's in line with looking at the body as a whole, looking for those connections, in order to experience better health. That includes weight loss.

If you are a menstruating female, you'll also want to make sure that your body is able to eliminate excess estrogen hormones. Obese men, especially middle-aged and older, can have an unbalanced estrogen-to-testosterone ratio. You need to sleep well and to make sure that there are no issues with your thyroid. We discussed the fact that lowering high insulin levels will help with weight loss.[61]

The good news is that it's not as complicated as it seems. We have gone over how different organs can help heal or impede proper function, and how these connections influence your health.

YOUR LIVER

As you begin to make some basic changes, a lot of these issues start to clear on their own. Parts of the body help other parts to heal. For example, the liver and the kidneys help detoxify your body, as does your skin. They are all connected and work together to heal seemingly unrelated health issues.

Skin problems can be connected to the liver. As your liver becomes less burdened and can work better, it takes pressure off your kidneys, which act as filters for the blood. I often see in patients that as liver issues clear up, many skin issues often clear up as well.

The body has an amazing ability to heal itself if given the right natural support. Many of the biggest health challenges most patients have are due to chronic inflammation, which can come from a variety of problems. But many of them can be addressed by looking at these fundamental issues we have been talking about.

Speaking of the liver, let's consider another example of the importance of paying attention to the whole body and its functions, rather than just looking at one parameter. Many people have low levels of vitamin D, but often their lab numbers do not increase much when they are prescribed the usual amount of vitamin D.

You need a healthy liver and kidneys to help activate vitamin D that is ingested with foods or supplements. But there can be other causes for low levels of vitamin D. Sometimes it is the body's complex way of protecting itself in the presence of parathyroid tumors. In these cases, high blood calcium levels can serve as an indicator.

Taking vitamin D, which is oil-based, with meals that contain long-chain fatty acids, such as fish oils, helps the body to absorb it better.[62]

I mentioned that it is important not to have excess estrogen. Fat cells are not like the back closet in your house, used for storage and rarely opened. Fat cells remain active, constantly making estrogen and inflammatory compounds, among other things.

Estrogen and thyroid hormones can work in opposite ways. Thyroid hormones help convert fat into energy, for example, and estrogen helps turn calories into fat.[63,64,65] Increased cortisol levels suppress the production of testosterone and help convert whatever testosterone is available into a female hormone.[66,67,68]

A lot of patients have told me that after eating, they feel full and wish they had eaten less. Many say that they didn't realize they had put so much food in their belly. It's something most of us have gone through at some time or another.

In addition to leptin, fat cells produce a hormone called *adiponectin*. Adiponectin is needed for a lot of good reasons. For example, it helps to increase insulin sensitivity, increase oxidation of fatty acids, reduce triglyceride levels, and improve glucose metabolism.

Higher adiponectin levels can decrease the risks of cancer. Guess what an elevated level of cortisol does to adiponectin? It reduces levels of that hormone.

Let's take a moment to review some of the topics we've discussed. I do this periodically throughout the book because research has shown that a review helps a person to store facts into long-term memory. So does a good night's sleep!

- We discussed how a good digestive system, which includes the intestines and beneficial bacteria, is important, because it affects how food is metabolized. We said that this could affect your appetite levels, brain health, and propensity for diabetes.

- We talked about the adrenal glands, the ones that produce stress hormones, and then addressed excess estrogen hormones as having a strong influence on sugar cravings, levels of energy, and on sleeping patterns.
- I pointed out that the brain burns calories when you are asleep, as well as helping heal the stomach lining.
- We discussed how cortisol works in relation to weight and appetite. I explained that it can increase insulin levels, which can increase weight.
- I mentioned that cortisol increases blood sugar levels. Cortisol preferentially breaks down muscle, which is composed of amino acids. Those amino acids are metabolized in the liver to produce glucose, or sugar, in the blood for the body to use as energy.
- We discussed how insulin can affect inflammation levels and that lowering high insulin levels makes it easier to lose fat.[69,70,71,72]
- We looked at how an increase in cortisol levels can contribute to an increase in high blood pressure, since cortisol constricts arteries. It's one reason why people under stress often see their blood pressure go up.[73,74,75,76]

Since we have been discussing weight loss, it's a good time to talk about childhood obesity.

Here's something to think about: when it comes to childhood obesity, what do the numbers 15 and 80 billion have in common?

What You Can Do Now

- Stand instead of sitting, take the stairs instead of the elevator, park a little farther away . . .
- Lose fat, not muscle. As you get older, incorporating weightlifting into your exercise routine becomes more and more important to help to maintain and build muscle mass.
- Too busy to make it to the gym? Try doing several series of 30 seconds of high-intensity exercise alternating with a minute of rest. Another form of high-intensity interval exercise is the Tabata protocol (http://tabataexercise.com) created by Dr. Izumi Tabata, which involves periods of high-intensity exercise and rest for a total of four minutes.
- Eat small high-protein snacks throughout the day if you feel weak or start getting irritated before meals. Protein keeps sugar levels, and serotonin, more stable. It also helps to increase muscle mass when followed by the right type of exercises.
- Make sure that all detoxifying and eliminatory organs and tissues are working well before starting a

weight-loss program, since problems here will affect how easily your body can handle the stress of weight loss. Consult with a clinician as necessary.

[24]

Fat Children? Act Now!

LET'S START WITH the number 15. It's generally considered the age when the number of fat cells in a person's body stops increasing.[1] That's an approximate age; the range is anywhere from 13 to 18, depending on the study.

I've seen a growing number of overweight children in my clinic. Many of them are teenagers with abnormal cholesterol levels, as well as abnormal liver enzymes. It is an epidemic. In the past 30 years, the percentage of children who are overweight has tripled.[2]

More than one-third of all children in America are now either obese or overweight.[3]

It's really a tragedy. In America, one out of every 10 children now has fatty liver disease. It used to be something that usually only adults had. The problem with fatty liver disease is that it can lead to more serious problems in the liver, including cirrhosis, which is not reversible.[4]

The title of this chapter urges parents to act now because children don't have the luxury of waiting to lose weight, as adults do, without experiencing important consequences, some of which are permanent.

The bodies of children of that age, perhaps up to age 18 or so, are different from adults in a number of ways, but especially when it comes to the issue of obesity.

And that's where the number 80 billion comes in.

Our fat cells are active hormonal agents, doing much more than just storing fat. For now, let's talk about the number of fat cells in an adult, which is approximately 80 billion. Don't confuse the number of fat cells with their size, though. As you gain weight, fat cells grow to many times their normal size.[5]

So why is it so important for children to lose the weight sooner rather than later?

There's a good reason, and if you have obese or overweight children, you need to act now. It has to do with how the body develops as a child and as an adolescent, specifically in regard to the number of fat cells.

For all of us, when we are young, the number of fat cells begins to grow and then plateaus. In adolescents, that happens between the ages of 13 and 20, depending on the study.[6] Many of these studies agree that if a child is overweight or obese during this critical time, when the number of fat cells increases, by the time he reaches adulthood he will have more fat cells than his normal-weight childhood friends.[7,8]

This high number of fat cells affects overweight children when they become adults, because people with a greater number of fat cells have a more difficult time losing weight than those with fewer fat cells.

Concerned parents often ask me, if their child loses the weight when she is an adult, won't those extra fat cells go away?

Unfortunately, no. The child's fat cells will shrink in size as she loses weight as an adult, but the number is set during adolescence by a number of factors, including genetics. However, childhood obesity plays a large role in determining the permanent number of fat cells, which children will have for the rest of their lives.

Taking Action

At what age does this all start? When do parents have to become concerned?

Now!

Parents need to start focusing on this as early as kindergarten. That's when weight patterns can begin to settle in for life. The greatest change in the percentage of children with obesity takes place by the time they are in the third grade.[9,10]

A number of parents think they're doing their children a favor by pampering them and making them feel more satisfied by giving them sugar and junk food. Instead, they're helping to set an unfortunate weight pattern for life, along with other metabolic consequences.

It's a tough problem to solve. If children are obese by the time they are 13, they usually stay obese for the rest of their childhood, and often as adults. The best time for parents to take action is before kindergarten. It's best to stop the weight gain before it becomes a pattern. Once the child is overweight or obese, by the time he or she starts school, it's possible, but quite hard, to reverse the trend, according to research.[11,12] Genetics plays a role, but we are not sure to what extent. However, a lot of it has to do with the weight of the mother during pregnancy and lactation. Keep in mind that families eat out of the same proverbial plate. That is, they eat the same types of foods and develop the same eating habits.

Those eating habits that the child is learning at the table of parents who are overweight usually will contribute to his or her obesity, or else the parents would have likely lost their excess weight by that point.

If a pregnant woman eats too much fat in her diet, her children as well as grandchildren might have an increased risk of breast cancer. Even if she has a son, the son might pass along the increased risk to his daughter, although he might be of normal weight.[13,14,15,16] I note this in the context that a balanced amount of healthy dietary fats is important in every diet, especially in pregnancy.

Pregnancy and Obese Children

Pregnant mothers who are overweight or obese tend to have babies who are fatter and also have more fat in their liver. This association has also been seen with fathers who were overweight or obese during conception. The trend is for these babies to have higher incidences of metabolic disorders in their life.[17,18]

The reasons are still being looked into, but there are indications that women who eat a high-fat diet during the last part of their pregnancy might have children with altered function, including issues with insulin sensitivity, in that part of the brain that helps control metabolism and appetite—the hypothalamus.[19] Additionally, it has been found that babies of obese mothers have different bacterial compositions in their gut compared with babies of mothers with normal weight.

Keep in mind that other stresses during pregnancy can have a big effect on how healthy a child will be. Remember that we talked about cortisol as the stress hormone in your body? Pregnant women who are under a lot of emotional stress, especially in the third trimester, produce higher levels of cortisol than normal. Research shows that this can lead to the child's having a greater risk of developmental and emotional issues.[20,21,22]

Additionally, women who experience depression while pregnant can give birth to children with a fourfold increase in the likelihood of developing depression.[23,24]

As you can see, there are a lot of factors during pregnancy that can have a marked effect on one's health as a child and during adulthood.

If you have or know of children with behavior problems, you may be interested in research showing that supplementation with omega-3 oils has been of help for aggressive and antisocial behavior problems. These types of oils help our brain cells to develop and function. In fact, our brain is composed of approximately 60 percent fat.

A study involving children from ages 8 to 16 who took one gram of omega-3s for six months showed a decrease in antisocial and aggressive behavior during that time and for another six months after they stopped taking the omega-3 supplements, an effect that was not seen in the control group. The study did not go beyond one year, however, it is suggestive of the role that omega-3s may play in childhood and possibly adult behavior.[25]

As far as whether genetics or the environment plays the main role in childhood obesity, it is interesting to note that wealthier families typically have fewer obese children. So do very poor families.

Most parents of obese children, including many with blood lab test results showing metabolic challenges such as fatty liver, view those children as being in good health, according to a recent study.[26]

If they are obese, why do most of their parents think they are healthy? Here is a big, and surprising, clue: half of the parents of obese children think their children are at a normal weight.[27]

This adds evidence to my initial point at the beginning of this book—that changing how you see yourself and your health, the big picture, is the most important step toward improving your health. This applies to how you look at your children as well. We need to change how we view things, to see them for what they really are at deeper levels, including finding the relationships, or connections, between you, your mind, your body, and the world around you.

Beyond the clinical data that I've shared with you, my sense is that expanding your viewpoint is the most important step you can take to secure better health for yourself and your loved ones. It is the basis, the foundation of health and life because it drives what you think and do—how you will respond to the challenges of illness and your environment.

Childhood obesity can be helped through physical exercise. Most parents are not involved enough in making sure that their obese children are exercising. After children are past the age of 14, it becomes harder for parents to instill the habit of exercise in their offspring.[28]

Research shows one method that does help children to lose weight, and it can be implemented immediately and without financial cost, although they will usually not be happy about it: reduce their television and computer time.[29]

The children in one study, when given access to a home computer between the fifth and eighth grades, experienced a persistent decline in math and reading scores. The weaker the children's reading and writing skills, the worse their scores became. They used their computer to surf the Internet, play games, and engage in social media rather than using it as a study tool.[30]

This is in line with what we discussed earlier about simply moving around more during the day to increase the body's metabolic rate and to burn more calories.

Childhood Obesity and Mental Health

There is an important connection, or association, between obesity and future psychiatric illnesses for kids. Obese children, and many overweight children, typically have high levels of an inflammatory chemical messenger known as *interleukin-6,* or IL-6. This can be checked with a simple blood test.

Nine-year-olds with the highest levels of IL-6 were approximately 50 percent more likely to be diagnosed with depression at age 18 than nine-year-olds with the lowest levels. The research also shows that the ones with the highest IL-6 levels at age nine are almost twice as likely to have a psychotic experience at age 18.[31]

The presence of higher-than-normal levels of inflammatory markers such as IL-6 or C-reactive protein increases the risk of developing type 2 diabetes.[32,33]

Helping your children to stay at a healthy weight level and to decrease inflammation at an early age can also give them a better chance of not suffering from depression or psychosis when they enter adulthood.

Helping Children to Lose Weight

There's a lot of good information out there regarding healthy foods. You already know most of it, but let me add something else that recent research has shown to help children who struggle with obesity. Sixteen-year-olds who get fewer than six hours of sleep have a 20 percent higher risk of being obese by the age of 21 than those who sleep eight hours or more.[34]

You can also give your child a glass of grapefruit juice and green apples. The green apples help keep away disorders associated with obesity by aiding the balance of healthy bacteria in the intestines.[35]

A glass of grapefruit juice a day, which has only 76 calories, might slow weight gain by as much as 20 percent among those who eat a high-fat diet. Additionally, it can lower glucose, insulin, triglycerides, and fat levels in the blood. A study showed that grapefruit juice could lower sugar in the blood as effectively as the leading diabetes drug, metformin.[36] These natural aids can also help nondiabetic youths and adults.

Much of what I have already mentioned about weight loss for adults in previous chapters applies to children as well. Let's look at some connections that we should keep in mind when considering how to help children lose weight.

Research we discussed earlier demonstrates that children are more vulnerable to pesticides and toxins, and they could have more of these toxins stored in their tissues, pound for pound, than an adult.

We will explore more deeply in the next chapter the connections between weight loss and toxins, and what you need to know about them to help you lose weight and be healthier. Weight loss involves the release of toxins from fat cells, which tend to store toxins. Children's bodies may have to process this additional toxic load released from their fat cells as they lose weight, making the weight-loss process more difficult. It is a connection that is worth putting attention on, since toxins impede weight loss.

Next, we'll explore more ways to help your weight go down, by helping something else . . . go up!

What You Can Do Now

- Help your children to be slimmer and healthier when they become adults by not giving in to demands for junk food.
- Exercise is a habit best instilled when very young.
- Make sure that someone with a good clinical eye tells you whether or not your child is overweight; research shows that your loving eyes can lie!

- If you want to have a child and you are overweight, whether you are a man or a woman, the time to lose the weight is now, before conception.

- A gram of omega-3s a day has been shown to help reduce aggressive behavior in children.

- More computer time has been shown to decrease reading and writing skills in children. Reducing computer time also reduces obesity.

- If you have an obese child, consider a blood test for inflammatory markers discussed in this chapter. These tests are inexpensive. Increased levels of the markers during childhood lead to much greater chances of depression, diabetes, and psychosis in adulthood.

- Grapefruit juice and green apples are great for helping with weight loss and with reducing high fat and sugar levels in the blood; one study showed one glass of grapefruit juice a day to be as effective as the diabetic drug metformin.

[25]

When Health Goes Up, Weight Goes . . .

THE LONGER A person remains obese, the greater the risk of that person's death. In fact, a 30-year-old who is very obese has a 12-fold increase in mortality, compared with a 30-year-old of normal weight. Being overweight or obese is also associated with a lot of serious diseases, such as diabetes, heart disease, high blood pressure, arthritis, gallbladder problems, emotional issues, and some cancers.[1]

There is some good news, however. Let's explore a connection between walking and reduced mortality rates. Even among the obese, doing daily exercise equal to walking briskly for 20 minutes each day can reduce the risk of premature death somewhere between 16 and 30 percent.[2] For overweight or obese people who are unable to exercise, or simply want more help in reducing cardiovascular risks, taking 500 mg of vitamin C daily on a time-release basis is as effective as regular exercise. Vitamin C helps to reduce protein compounds in the blood that constrict blood vessels.

Let's go over some of the things we've touched on relating to weight loss.

- We explored the importance of feeling well to give ourselves a better chance of losing weight. We discussed how being overweight can be viewed as a consequence, as well as the importance of losing fat, not muscle.
- We talked about losing weight as an event that is stressful on the body, releasing toxins that your organs have to be ready to process and eliminate. We discussed how your thyroid function could slow down as you lose weight, as well as the importance of having good intestinal flora. Thyroid function, which is involved in burning calories, can be weaker when that stress hormone, cortisol, is high for too long.
- We covered chronic inflammation, high blood sugar, and high insulin levels that make it harder to lose fat and affect your appetite centers. We also talked about the effect of comfort food on your neurotransmitters and your brain, and how it makes you feel.
- We discussed how the effects of chronic stress create cortisol, making it harder for you to burn fat.
- We went over the benefits of creating daily habits of doing little things, like taking the stairs or sitting less, that would add up over time in helping you lose weight. We discussed the importance of acting now to address

weight issues in children—remember that you have a narrow time window—act now!

Fix the Body, Fix the Fat!

This brings us to the big picture for losing weight: in order to fix the fat, you need to fix the body!

Let's explore the topic of our appetite further, because for most people trying to lose weight, it's an important topic. In doing so, we will again revisit how functions in other parts of the body can affect one thing—in this case, your appetite.

We've talked about insulin and how it can affect your appetite, and I mentioned before that high levels make it harder for your body to burn fat. Let's make another connection now between insulin, your brain, and appetite.

According to research, your brain's cells include receptors of insulin that need to function well to control your appetite levels.[3] However, similar to when there is too much sugar for long periods in the blood, the brain cells can also become resistant to insulin.[4]

The insulin in the brain works in less defined ways than it does in the rest of your body. However, let's focus on what is important to know as it relates to weight. Abnormally high levels of insulin, in a condition known as *hyperinsulinemia,* not only increase appetite and the amount of food you eat, but they make you want to have more of the sugary stuff.

Another reason to keep the insulin levels down, and not just because of the threat of diabetes.

The liver is also involved in this process: it is the body's key metabolic organ—responsible, among other things, for helping store glucose, breaking down glycogen into glucose, and helping the body convert the digested sugars from your meals into triglycerides.

It's the reason why those who eat a lot of fatty foods or drink too much alcohol can develop a fatty liver. Sugary foods and refined carbohydrates are also associated with decreases in brain function and mood, including depression.[5] It's a tricky thing; I mentioned that eating carbohydrates can make you feel good by increasing temporary feel-good neurotransmitters, such as serotonin and dopamine. On the other hand, continuing to do that disrupts the brain's ability to create normal levels of those neurotransmitters.

Because people eat that way, over a period of time they're going to want to keep going back to the breads and sugary stuff to get a quick, feel-good boost, thus creating a vicious circle. Food eaten this way can act like coffee, which is a stimulant; however, it may also wear down the body's natural energy resources over time. It's one reason why many get addicted to those great cups of java.

You can see why getting off the breads and similar types of carbohydrates is pretty hard for a lot of people. It's not just about the taste, the sugar boost, or having something to fill their stomach; rather, they have been relying on these types of high-energy, fatty foods to help modulate the neurotransmitters in their brain, which change how they feel.

My sense is that, on a deep level, success in losing weight for most people is really about being able to successfully handle their feelings and moods without eating the typical mood-altering foods. When consuming too much sugar, the liver is burdened; for example, triglycerides, a type of fat, are deposited in the liver as fat and lower its function. Keep in mind that the liver performs over 500 functions and is a key organ for good health.

An increase in liver fat content has been shown to predict type 2 diabetes and increase insulin resistance.[6,7,8] Almost half of all the insulin produced by the pancreas is used by the liver, usually within 10 minutes. The kidneys take up a good amount of the remaining insulin.[9]

Beyond Exercise and Eating Well

Exercise and eating well are important parts of any sound weight-loss or health program. However, as we discussed, research shows that most people who tried a food and exercise program to lose weight ended up gaining the weight back within months. On a level of personal experience, ask yourself how many diet plans you or your friends have been on in your life.

That's why we need to help support the body systems naturally, so that as the body's functions begin to work normally, you will naturally feel more energy. Your body works well when it is prepared to handle the physiological stress of losing weight; then it becomes an important friend in helping you to lose weight while feeling well, with good energy, and not going hungry.

As a result, you will feel more motivated to exercise and will get even more benefit from it. I have had patients tell me that they felt so weak after doing exercise during a weight-loss program that they ended up eating high-caloric foods because they wanted to quickly feel better again.

That's why we need to take an expanded view of all the body processes and to help them, naturally, as a first step to losing the inches.

Improve the way your body functions, because that makes it easier for you to make better lifestyle choices, and later the image in the mirror changes.

As I said, fix the body to fix the fat!

With that in mind, would you like to change the shape of the image in your mirror to your liking by . . . eating chocolate every day?

What You Can Do Now

- A quick, 20-minute daily walk helps decrease rates of premature death for obese people by up to 30 percent. Go for a walk every day!
- Getting high insulin levels down will make you feel less hungry. Controlling your sugar levels helps to control your appetite.
- Fix the body to fix the fat!
- Handle your moods to handle your weight. Handle your weight to handle your moods.

  Many people are overweight because of their relationship to food and how they feel about the emotions they are experiencing. Many people are much more uncomfortable than others when it comes to feeling certain emotions and will use food to suppress them. Others use alcohol, drugs, anger, and other emotional avoidance behaviors. I will mention again that counseling, including free cognitive behavior therapy online, such as with MoodGYM, can be helpful (https://moodgym.anu.edu.au/welcome).

[26]

Eating Chocolate to Lose Weight!

REMEMBER THAT WE spoke about an emotional component to food, how it modulates the function of our brain to make us feel better? That's why it's so hard to stop eating certain things. Even when we know they aren't good for us. This happens especially when we're under stress.

How do you feel, really feel, when you bite into a piece of warm, dark, luscious chocolate?

And how do you feel when you start a diet, knowing that you will be facing pounds and pounds of broccoli, fish, spinach, and other non-fun stuff for weeks or months?

Most people don't get the warm fuzzies at the thought of starting a new diet. Who in their right mind would? They usually begin by pumping themselves up, looking for motivation by reminding themselves that they can't go on like this, squeezing into ever-tighter jeans and dresses, and knowing that they just have to do it, to make a commitment.

Despair has started most diets, and frustration has broken more diets than we could ever count.

We know what happens to most people on diets, right? We've already looked at national as well as global numbers, 188 countries, and they're not good.

What if you knew that on every day of your diet you could have fun food, food that made you feel good? Food that tasted so good, you could use it as a reward for having followed your plan that day? Wouldn't that make it easier to stick to your diet?

I'm talking about eating chocolate every day. Sometimes two or three times daily!

I've seen it work, and I'm suggesting that it's something you can experiment with. Have just a bite before or after dinner. Half an ounce of dark chocolate is fine. But eat it slowly, let it melt in your mouth, and be aware of it as it happens.

If this sounds like a screenplay for a *Star Wars* movie and that I am suggesting that you be one with the chocolate, you're half right. Half an ounce of dark chocolate isn't much, so you really want to eat it slowly, to enjoy it. Make sure that you are, as Obi-Wan might say, one with the cocoa!

Spend a couple of wonderful minutes savoring it. It's not much calorie-wise—around 75 calories. Really not much when you add up the calories you eat in a day. If you're stuck on having these extra calories added, jump rope for a few minutes. That will burn them off.

Many stores sell these chocolates in little containers, prepackaged. For example, you could have one Hershey's Kiss before and after lunch, and then the same at dinner, and you're still at around 85 calories of chocolate for the day.

Why eat chocolate before a meal?

It's a good question, and a curious thing. When you eat chocolate before you have a meal, your brain and body feel so satisfied with that little sweet bit that you might find yourself not wanting to eat as much as you usually do.

Try it. I speak from experience. It's worked for others who have lost weight more pleasantly. I have been suggesting that you look at your health from a different perspective.

That's a sweet example!

We've also explored the need to seek new viewpoints, to approach our health with an expanded sense of inquiry, patients and physicians alike. I think that part of this new view includes being easy on ourselves in ways that are good for us.

We recognize that life is often challenging and can be quite stressful. Then we add the physiological and emotional stress of a diet, which can be tough.

We need more practitioners, whether doctors, dietitians, or nutritional specialists, to keep in mind the importance of accounting for our emotions and for how our brain really functions when it comes to losing weight. We shouldn't add an emotional obstacle course to an already restrictive food plan.

It's not just a pleasure dynamic that I'm talking about. A study showed that consuming up to 100 grams of chocolate daily was associated with a 25 percent decreased risk of death and 11 percent lower risk of cardiovascular disease, compared with risks for people who didn't eat chocolate.[1]

Most people enjoy having a piece of chocolate. It contains biological compounds that make us feel better and helps release feel-good endorphins and neurotransmitters. It has magnesium, which is why some women crave chocolate before their menstruation, and heart-protective effects if you eat chocolate containing 85 percent cocoa or more. At that level, the bitterness, which we talked about, can serve as a digestive aid. But if it's too bitter, try some with less cocoa content.

Research points to an association of milk chocolate, not just dark chocolate, with reduced cardiovascular issues. The point is to enjoy it. So why not?

Healthy Brain, Healthy Food Choices

There's another reason why I suggest doing something like this. It has to do with the way our brain functions.

To put it simply, the anterior part of the front of our brain is known as the *prefrontal cortex*. It is what we use to make plans and decisions and to reason. It's what we use to stop reaching for junk food when we're on a diet and what we use in choosing not to engage in behavior that's not in our best interests. In other words, the prefrontal cortex helps us to control our impulses.

It's important to have a healthy brain to make better food choices.

The rest of our brain, and I'm speaking in general terms, is where a lot of our impulses and desires arise from. The front of our brain is like the adult holding back the kid—the back of our brain—who wants to eat everything in life's proverbial candy store.

The front of our brain thinks things through and takes time and consequences into account. The emotional, impulsive parts live only in the moment, wanting pleasure and satisfaction now.

Often it can feel like a struggle within you, and doubtless it has. You are tempted to do something for immediate pleasure, but another part of you knows that in the long run it's not going to serve you well. For many, it starts with the first action in the morning. Do you ignore the alarm clock and enjoy the pleasure of staying in bed, or do you get up, shower, have breakfast, and make sure you get to work on time?

That's the decision-making part of your brain trying to work things out with the impulsive part, trying to reach a compromise. Sometimes the reasoning part of your brain wins, but other times you end up with a bagel and cream cheese in your mouth that you later regret. That goes for almost every type of choice in your life, not just food.

Now here is where it gets really interesting, since this ties into a number of regretful choices that we might have made in our lives, including our food choices.[2,3] When you feel mentally tired, research shows that it's easier to make poor choices. It's not just confined to foods; even judges have been found to make less favorable decisions before their recess. The term for it is *decision fatigue*.[4]

It's one reason why I have been stressing how important it is to be healthy and to feel well in order to lose weight more easily. Otherwise, our tired brain will make it an easier choice to reach for the potato chips, bagels, candy, sugary drinks, or whatever our particular mood-and-energy-altering gastronomic product of choice is.

We all have our little quirks. It's a big factor. It sabotages so many well-intended food programs.

So where does the blessed chocolate come in? There are times when the pace of life can make us feel tired or stressed. That's when it's more tempting to eat badly. So it's good to know that you can have some chocolate at some point. And it doesn't have to be chocolate—it can be a little of whatever you like.

I mentioned chocolate and its effects on your brain's neurotransmitters, those specialized messenger molecules. Genetic testing reveals a variation in some people that could put them more at risk for emotional eating.[5,6]

Emotional eating is closely associated with the levels of certain neurotransmitters, such as dopamine and serotonin. Chocolate helps with maintaining good levels of these neurotransmitters, and so do avocado and the herb rhodiola, among other things.

Foods that are naturally rich in B vitamins, fish oil, magnesium, and the amino acid tyrosine can be useful. I mentioned the use of audiovisual brainwave synchronization devices as well.

Most people eat out of habit, because of the way that food can change how they feel. Diet is as much about working with moods and feelings as it is about calorie counting.

When people are happy and feel good, it's easier for them to stay away from what they know isn't good for them or their weight.

There is interesting research that shows just how strong an effect certain foods have on us—sometimes even addictive effects. One study involved Oreo cookies, which have a creamy filling between two chocolate wafers.

Like many, when I indulge, I usually eat the filling first.

It turns out that there is a scientific basis for this habit. Laboratory rats, when given a choice between cocaine and Oreo cookies, usually choose the cookies. Researchers have found that the part of the brain that is associated with pleasure and reward was more strongly activated by the cookies than by cocaine![7]

It's the combination of sugar and fat, it seems, that makes the cookies so attractive. And, not to mention, they have chocolate.

Guess how the rats ate the Oreos? Just like you and me. They ate the white filling first.

Between bugs in the gut that control food cravings, which we discussed, and cookies packing a stronger punch than hard-core drugs, no wonder it's a challenge for people to keep the weight off!

In truth, a lot of things push us in the direction of weight gain. But there are also a lot of things we can do to counteract this that come naturally and effortlessly to us when we are healthy and feeling well.

We've been talking about what to do to change our image in the mirror. We have covered the fact that you need to fix the body to fix the weight; that being overweight is a consequence, like an image in a mirror. And that we need to make changes inwardly because being obese is a reflection of our internal body processes.

A lot of people start feeling bad when they start a diet. There are a number of reasons for this, one being that the systems in your body have to be fairly healthy and strong to handle weight loss well. Most people's systems aren't ready to begin so smoothly.

Weight Loss Is Traumatic!

Believe it or not, weight loss is a traumatic event for the body.

Burning your fat stores releases a number of toxins into the bloodstream as the fat cells shrink in size. Toxins circulating in your body, whether from external sources or internally released, cause cellular damage. Injury to the cells and tissue of your body constitutes one definition for trauma.

If your body's detoxifying and elimination channels, such as your liver, gallbladder, kidneys, and intestines, aren't working well, it will be harder for you to feel well while undergoing a weight-loss program, making it more difficult to be successful over the long run.[8]

Your body might simply not be ready to lose the weight because it cannot handle well the increased toxic load.

People who lose weight often have increased levels of toxins in their blood, such as organochlorines, which include PBCs, or *polychlorinated biphenyls,* found in common household products. The fat cells release them as you lose weight. These are toxic environmental agents that can negatively affect how your hormones and organs work.[9] That includes your thyroid, which acts as a calorie-burning metabolic regulator.

Your liver and gallbladder need to be happy and working well in order to metabolize toxins. For menstruating women, the liver helps break down the female hormones associated with the end of their previous menstrual cycle and prepares the body for the next cycle. If your liver and body don't do this well enough, it can lead to premenstrual symptoms.

The liver and the gallbladder also work together to release these metabolites into your intestines, so your intestines need to be working well. If not, these toxic byproducts might be reabsorbed into your blood again. This includes hormones that your liver has already spent energy to break down.[10,11]

As you can see, helping yourself to lose weight by getting rid of toxins is not just about one thing, such as a body part, working well; rather, it's about systems working together. It's about interrelationships. Your kidneys also work to help eliminate toxins. So do your lungs and your skin, for that matter. They work together.

Therefore, for optimal detoxification and elimination of these toxins from your body, among other things, you shouldn't be constipated or have intestinal permeability—another name for leaky gut.

You want the digested food remnants, as well as toxic metabolites processed by your liver, to be moved out of your body. You don't want them to be reabsorbed at the end of your intestines because of permeability issues, such as those associated with a leaky gut.

Working Together

Other aspects of your body need to work well to help you lose weight.

Your adrenals need to be working well because when you are eating less and watching what you eat, you will be eating sugary substances less often. In between meals, the brain will depend in part on the adrenals to make sure there are adequate fuel levels in the blood, day or night.

It will be important to have stable sugar levels, because without them you might have more difficulty maintaining normal levels of feel-good neurotransmitters in your brain. Without proper levels of these neurotransmitters, you might want to reach for a slice of pizza or a bag of potato chips to give you a quick mood boost.

Having a good supply of oxygen to your brain will also be important to keep you mentally alert.

Anemia, which I have seen in the blood tests of many menstruating women who experienced heavy bleeding, can lead to a decrease in the amount of oxygen to the brain. As a result, you can end up experiencing brain fatigue, which can lead to symptoms, or consequences, such as having trouble focusing, or dizziness. People often eat sugary foods to try to compensate.

Remember, it's when we don't feel good that we typically break out of our hard-won healthy eating patterns: decision fatigue.

Water

Our thirst mechanism starts to slow down in our 20s, so we have to remember to drink even though we aren't thirsty. As an adult, if you get thirsty during the course of the day, it usually means you probably should have drunk water some time ago. There are other reasons for it as well; diabetics and people with congestive heart failure, among others, can be thirstier than normal.[12,13,14,15,16]

Water helps reduce toxic concentration levels in your body and helps the body to have better and more frequent bowel movements. Decreased toxin levels help you to lose weight more easily. Additionally, if you drink 16 ounces of water half an hour before eating, it has been shown to make a significant difference in helping you to lose weight and to keep it off. One of the ways that it helps is to signal stretch receptors in the stomach that take some time to inform the brain that the stomach is full—kind of like filling the car quickly with gas until it overflows but the gas tank marker takes longer to show full. People who drink the 16 ounces one-half hour before a meal eat 20 percent less food. Try doing this with low-calorie soup, and it's a home run, because the brain is also informed that nutrients are already on board before you sit down to eat.[17,18]

My suggestion is to drink very little water with meals, if you can. Drink water half an hour before a meal, as suggested above, and wait a couple of hours after you finish a meal to drink again. The less water you drink during meals, the more you will chew. Many health practitioners feel that drinking too much water while eating can interfere with digestion.[19]

Many people think they should be drinking water most of the day to keep hydrated. As in nature, everything, including water intake, is best if done in balance, with the right timing.

You might remember that we discussed the importance of having good acid levels in your stomach, not just for digestion but also to help kill pathogens. You want levels that are not too high or too low, and want the acids to be produced at the right time.

Think of using that same perspective with water. There is a connection between acid levels and water.

Proper acid levels in our stomach act as a sentry against bacteria and help with digestion.[20] When you drink too much water, it sharply dilutes these beneficial acid levels. It dilutes them as strongly as antacid prescriptions, and more quickly. It just does so for less time.[21]

That means drinking water during meals decreases the potency of the acid in your stomach, which is critical for digestion of food. This dilution weakens the acid's ability to protect you from harmful agents in the food, such as *H. pylori, E. coli,* salmonella, and others.[22,23]

It is hard to overemphasize the importance of chewing your food well. When I ask many of my patients who complain of digestive issues how well they chew their food, they admit to eating quickly.

What You Can Do Now

- Eat half an ounce of chocolate slowly before lunch and dinner. Yeah! Another reason why we have to work hard to save this planet. It's the only one with chocolate!

- Don't go to the supermarket, to a restaurant, or to a dinner party when you are hungry. Pre-eat, even if it's just a couple of hundred calories, preferably with high-protein content. Spoil your appetite, not your figure! Don't sit down to eat when you are hungry!

- Drink 16 ounces of water, or have a large bowl of soup, one-half hour before lunch and/or dinner.

You can add fiber to the water. Alternatively, eat something that has protein, just a hundred or so calories, 30 minutes before a meal. Research shows that you will eat around 20 percent less food. That's about four pounds a month lost right there!

[27]

Just Chew It!

MANY PEOPLE THINK chewing is not important as long as we get the food down, often with water. Let's focus on saliva, because it's an often-neglected part of good digestion.

Your body can produce up to half a gallon of saliva each day. Saliva helps your body to begin digestion, particularly for some carbohydrates and, to a more limited extent, fats. Saliva has antiviral and antibacterial properties and helps protect your mouth and esophagus.[1,2,3,4,5]

So, as you can see, water cannot replace saliva. What else is important to your health about chewing?

Chewing helps the production of saliva in your mouth. One of the advantages to chewing your food and juices well is that it prepares them better for digestion. It helps your digestive system work more easily and efficiently. In fact, we are built to chew a lot! The main chewing muscles, known as the *masseter* muscles, are the strongest muscles for their size in our body.

Keep in mind that when you chew well, it means that you are eating more slowly, which helps you to eat less because there are mechanical receptors in your stomach that inform your brain how much food you have eaten. But the message takes a while to get there.

So chewing each mouthful more times not only brings out the flavor in each bite, helps digestion, and helps kill bugs in your food, but also helps your brain to become more aware that you are full, more quickly. And it helps activate nerve centers in the brain to prepare the body for digestion. Yes, there is also an important connection between your starting to eat food, your brain, and good digestion. Consider chewing softer foods a minimum of 10 times before swallowing. For harder food, chewing up to 30 times would be helpful.

I lived and practiced in Sardinia, a beautiful island west of Rome, a number of years ago. There I met a couple at a dinner party. Overlooking white sandy beaches and the pristine waters that Sardinia is famous for, the man happily remarked that he had lost over 100 pounds without feeling any hunger pangs, and usually eating until he felt full. His wife vouched for him, saying that it had taken a couple of years but that she saw him patiently chewing anything that was not water 20 times before swallowing, including soups.

I remember many years ago walking into an organic restaurant in Berkeley, California, and seeing a carved wooden sign above a doorway. It read: *Happy is the man who chews well.*

Many people experience bloating and gas after eating. This can often be a result of eating quickly and not chewing well. If you eat too quickly, you might have a feeling about 20 minutes later that you overate and are uncomfortably full.

In a digestive nutshell, these are two good reasons why you want to chew well: to help increase your overall health and to lose weight.

Your Thyroid and Weight Loss

We've been talking about losing weight, the challenges people face in doing so, and what they can do about it. Remember that I said people who lose weight often release toxins into their bloodstream?

We've illustrated through examples how the body is connected in ways that seem distant but really have effects that make a difference to our health. In this case, let's make a connection between your fat cells and your thyroid as you try to lose weight, and discuss how it can make weight loss more difficult.

When the fat cells shrink during weight loss, a number of toxins are released. These toxins have an effect on your thyroid gland. Your thyroid gland helps to control how many calories you are burning off during the day. When you lose weight, the toxins released decrease your resting metabolic rate and can decrease the level of the active thyroid hormone known as T3 in your body.

Here's the kicker: if you have increased toxins in your blood that are being released from fat cells, and those toxins decrease your resting metabolic rate, your fat-burning rate, that makes it harder to lose weight!

Weight loss can affect your active thyroid hormone levels, which are necessary for a number of other functions, including having a healthy and well-functioning digestive system.

That's another example of how the body is connected like a spider web. You cannot disturb one part of it without feeling the effects throughout the web.

It's easy to see more clearly why it is so important to be as healthy as you can and to have your systems working well before you embark on a weight-loss program. You want to be able to choose a program that your body can handle, one that gives you a better chance of sticking to it.

Gain It to Lose It

To lose weight, you first have to gain health. Everything in life, including the laws of nature, works in balance. Think of it as children playing on a seesaw. As one side goes up, the other goes down. It's easier, when you increase your health, to decrease your weight.

It works the other way around, too.

The less healthy you are, the easier it is to gain weight. One way a lot of people experience this is when they don't have much energy, don't sleep well, and feel stressed. That's when many find it more difficult to resist eating foods they know aren't good for them.

Some people who are on a weight-loss program and whose body was not ready actually feel better in the short term, when they go back to eating junk or high-carbohydrate food. One reason is that by getting off the diet, they stop their fat cells from shrinking and therefore from releasing more toxins into their bodies—toxins that they couldn't process and eliminate well.

There's more to this than any one book could cover. That's why developing the habit of thinking through the issues with whatever information you have on hand and asking the right questions—like the story of the young doctor in India who first had to ask the right questions in order to receive the right information—is one of the most important things you can do for your health and for your life.

When it comes to eating food, as with the varying ways in which people respond to drugs, we have different bodies and respond differently. However, there are some general guidelines that work well for most people. There is some flexibility here, so you need to adapt what works best for you as well as for your family.

The Best Food Plan in the World!

Would you like to know what the best food plan is for you, from all the thousands of possible food plans in the world?

It's the food plan that you are able and willing to follow! It makes no sense to design nutritional or exercise strategies that are beyond the reach of your present level of health, or of your inclination. It's a sure-fire way to have perhaps short-term success but likely long-term failure—and frustration.

We need to be practical and start with small, easy steps. As your health improves, you'll find it easier to make healthier food choices in the long run.

When people think of food plans at some point, their attention is usually focused on calories. Are all calories alike? Unlike the aphorism "A rose, is a rose, is a rose," not all calories are the same when it comes to your weight!

Just because a food substance is *isocaloric,* meaning it has the same number of calories as another food substance, doesn't mean it is isometabolic. In other words, it might not have the same metabolic effects regarding your weight.[6] Different types of food that have the same amount of calories might affect your body differently and might have an influence on your attempts to lose fat.

For example, if you eat a product made with fructose, a common sweetener, it sends the brain a weaker signal that you are full than if you eat a product with the same amount of calories of another type of sugar, glucose.

Research indicates that fructose, found in many soft drinks and other types of sweet foods, might actually stimulate hunger. It also causes other health concerns, including insulin resistance, that go beyond its caloric effect.[7,8,9,10,11,12]

We know that eating the same amount of calories, or even the same foods, at different points in our life, depending on the circumstances, can have different effects on our propensity to develop diabetes, obesity, and inflammation.[13,14]

The amount of calories in foods cannot always be taken as an absolute; rather, it should be taken in context. A one-dimensional approach limits our healing potential, whether we are talking about a prescription or even food.

Here is another example of how the condition of our entire organism, including our emotions, can affect how our body responds to a meal. If a woman has a stressful incident and the next day eats just one high-fat comfort meal, she will slow her metabolic rate for seven hours after that meal, when compared with someone who also ate that high-fat meal but hadn't been stressed.

If you make eating high-fat foods after stress a habit, as many do, it adds pounds of fat each year.[15]

There's more. In this type of situation, the high-fat meal also increases insulin levels more than usual. If there is a history of depression, even if the woman was not depressed that day, the usual amount of fat (triglycerides) in her blood will also increase more than usual.

Eating and Emotions

Sometimes patients share with me, at times with a sense of shame, that they think of food as a good friend who is always there. They might argue with someone, or feel disappointed with their friends, their family, or people at work. But the taste of food, and how it makes them feel, is always consistent. It never lets them down and is always there for them.

Unhealthy eating is a big challenge for so many to overcome. We talked about how food influences our brain. That's what makes it so tough. Emotional habits associated with food choices are a big reason why people have a hard time losing weight.

Professional counseling might be the best choice for some people when they become aware of this and can't seem to break the habit. Talking to a friend about it or writing in a diary when dieting might also work well.

I have talked to people who have deep insights into the nature of the mind-body, as well as the body-mind, connection. Some of them feel that any time you undergo a cleansing, detoxification, or significant weight loss, it's helpful to look for what else in your life needs to shift, balance, or release. Look for connections that go beyond physical issues.

The suggestion is that physical changes are processed best when they are integrated with mental and emotional changes. A wise insight is to consider what other life patterns, besides changing the shape of our body, also need changing. Some of the time, it's simply about changing how we see ourselves and what's around us.

In that vein, let's explore the connections between the foods you eat, weight, and better health from a different point of view: food grouping.

Glycemic Load vs. Glycemic Index—and a Hidden Connection

Food can be grouped in a variety of ways. For example, foods that are high in different types of sugar are considered to have a *high-glycemic-index* score. High-glycemic-index foods stimulate insulin production by the body and decrease fat burning. The higher the score, the more the food type does this.

The glycemic food index is the most commonly known index, but if you search the Internet, you will find information on other indexes, such as the glycemic load and insulin indexes, that are more useful.

The glycemic load index is a composite measure of the glycemic index and the total amount of carbs in a food. At the end of the day, the total number of carbs consumed is important to your blood sugar levels and health. I recommend that you spend some time looking at these indexes. It won't take long. They will help guide you in making better food choices.

Generally speaking, for you and your family, it's best to eat foods that are low on the glycemic load or insulin indexes. That works for most people, especially if you want to lose weight.

Whichever index you use, you want to choose foods that decrease sugar and insulin levels in the blood. Eating foods with lower glycemic load levels will lower your fat levels and shrink those love handles. That is especially important for your health, not just your body shape. Fat around your waist is the worst of all for your health. I mentioned in chapter 6 that excess belly fat leads to greater risk of cardiovascular issues and makes it harder for your pancreas to work well. Eating low-glycemic-load foods can be helpful. Substituting good fats for carbohydrates will reduce your insulin response.

So far, it seems pretty straightforward: eat less of foods with a higher total sugar content to decrease your blood sugar response after meals. In chapter 15 we discussed the fact that a higher postprandial glucose response and its metabolic consequences were associated with a wide array of conditions, including obesity, hypertension, metabolic disease, cardiovascular problems, and diabetes.

So where's the hidden connection that I mentioned in the subheading? It's inside you—what else is new? What if you went to dinner with a friend and discovered that the healthy sushi that you dutifully limited yourself to increased your blood sugar more than your companion's meal did for her, even though she ate a cookie and ice cream?

It happens more than you think. It turns out that our blood sugar responses to meals vary quite a bit from person to person, and even within a person, depending on the circumstance.

There are a number of factors that affect how much your blood sugar will rise after a meal, and one of them is your gut microbiome. That's the collection of microbes in your intestinal tract. Unhealthy bacteria is associated with higher sugar levels, while healthy ones decrease them.[16,17]

This is a hidden connection to your sugar responses that you want to take advantage of. It's not just about what you eat, but also about how your internal environment responds to what you eat. In terms of sugar levels, what is OK to eat for one person may not be for someone else. Someone's "healthy food" may be the equivalent of junk food for someone else in terms of a sugar-level response.

Other factors that come into play with lowered sugar levels include your lifestyle, sleep, genetics, and previous meals.[18,19,20] In the future, my sense is that as these connections become more well-known, individualized eating plans will become common, taking a number of factors into consideration, and that stool samples will become a readily used part of constructing an individualized food program.

Let's spend some time talking about a favorite subject for a lot of food lovers: meals that contain fat. For over a couple of decades, we have been told to go on low-fat diets—that eating fats would increase our cholesterol and cause a number of other health issues. We know now that eating fats that are good for us is important to our health. Our brain is composed of approximately 60 percent essential fats. The liver, for example, manufactures approximately 75 percent of our cholesterol, even if we didn't eat anything that could raise it.

I remember going on a three-day water fast and seeing my cholesterol levels, which were at normal levels before the fast, rise at the end of the fast—before I resumed eating. In fact, they rose to red-flag levels in the blood-test results, according to the lab's parameters.

The body does this because cholesterol is necessary for many reasons. You need it to help manufacture sex hormones and to maintain healthy cell membranes, as well as for a number of other necessary body functions, including healing. Fasting accelerates healing cycles throughout the body and is a health tool that has been used for many thousands of years throughout the world.

A cholesterol level that is too low, to the surprise of many, is also not healthy.[20,21,22,23,24,25] In an Italian study, low cholesterol levels were associated with depression and suicide. Neither drought nor flood; everything necessary in balance.[26]

Fiber for Health and Weight Loss

To lose fat from the body, having adequate levels of high-quality protein along with fiber is important. The amount can vary from person to person. Eating protein helps suppress the appetite. It also takes more energy for your body to digest, which burns more calories. This is what's known as the *thermal effect,* which helps to increase the total number of calories that your body has burned in a day.

There is another benefit to making sure that you have enough fiber in your diet, which the average person does not. The bacteria in our intestines digest fiber, fermenting and releasing acetate. Scientists are discovering that acetate is an anti-appetite molecule that tells our brain to stop eating.[27]

You might remember that a few pages ago I mentioned research showing how drinking 16 ounces of water half an hour before each meal decreased the amount of calories people normally ate by 20 percent. Consider adding fiber to this water, as I suggest to many of my patients, for extra help in controlling your appetite, as well as for its many beneficial aspects to your digestive tract and your health.

Resistant Starches—the Third Type of Fiber

I mentioned soluble and insoluble fibers in the section on juicing. There is another type, known as *resistant starch,* that can help you to lose weight and to feel fuller despite eating the same amount of food.

Resistant starch is a type of carbohydrate found in seeds, unprocessed whole grains, high amylose corn starch, raw potatoes, green banana flour, and legumes, among others. Some portions of foods develop into resistant starches after being cooked and then refrigerated or cooled, such as bread and potatoes. It is not digested in the small intestine, reaching the large intestine, where it acts like fiber.

It's wise for many to consider adding natural resistant starch to their food, such as cassava starch, high-maize corn starch, and green banana flour. Raw potato starch has the advantage of being very low in digestible carbohydrates, which is great if you want to lose weight.

Often you can add these products to flours, cereal, and pastas. The starch helps to reduce the number of calories consumed, since it has between 50 and 75 percent of the calories found in flour and rapidly digested carbohydrates.[28] It increases the amount of good bacteria in your gut and makes good bowel movements easier.[29,30]

The cells in your colon use mostly short-chain fatty acids for energy. Resistant starch helps to produce a type of short-chain fatty acid, *butyrate,* which is the preferred source of energy for these cells and which helps to protect the colon from cancer and inflammation.[31]

Resistant starch may help to improve sensitivity to insulin.[32] However, while the benefits of resistant starch to the health of your gut are indisputable, research involving long-term insulin and glucose changes with resistant starch has not yet demonstrated consistent results.

I also mentioned that if you drastically reduce your calorie count during dieting, your body may make up for it later by reducing your resting metabolic rate, which helps to determine how many calories you burn in a day.

That's one reason why a number of patients who have lost a lot of weight quickly put it back on, and then some. Then they have a harder time losing weight down the road. An extreme diet could lead to a 20 percent reduction in calories burned throughout the course of a day. Yet others seem to do well with this type of approach, and some studies, including those noted here, point in the direction of this being a successful approach.

Most of us who want to lose weight would benefit by taking in around 500 calories less than what we are burning off each day—more if you are doing well and exercise a lot. You should check with your doctor first, as there are always exceptions. Charts are available on the Internet that can give you a sense of approximately how many calories you are burning in a typical day.

PROTEIN

On the subject of protein, let's explore how your body digests and assimilates it. I've noted that it can be a good aid to weight loss.

Protein is broken down and digested in the stomach, where it needs high enough levels of stomach acid to do so. Eating a lot of carbohydrates will slow protein digestion; try to limit your refined carbohydrates.[33]

Most of the digestion and assimilation of protein is carried out in the small intestine. Studies conducted with radio telemetry capsules indicated that the digestive tract stays acidic, except for a small section at the end of the small intestine. That means almost all digestion takes place in an acidic environment, despite alkaline secretions from glands into the small intestine, such as the pancreas.[34,35,36]

This is why it's important to have good levels of stomach acid, along with a healthy stomach, to help you digest your protein. But . . . you need a team!

You need the coordination and good function of other organs and glands, such as the pancreas and the small intestine, for digestion, and the liver to help put the end products of protein, amino acids, to good use.

With all the attention we have been placing on the stomach to help digest protein, as helpful as that is, it's the pancreas that is the biggest contributor to protein digestion.[37]

The elderly tend to produce less stomach acid, which is needed to digest protein. Research shows that for them the type of protein best absorbed by the body is not fish, chicken, or milk. It is a type of protein that a person can absorb more quickly, such as whey protein, which is also very low in lactose, less than 1 percent.[38] I mentioned earlier that supplementation with whey protein, taken over a six-month period, aided in the healing of the intestines for people suffering from irritable bowel disease.

To Eat or Not to Eat

A lot of people skip breakfast when attempting to lose weight. The thinking is that the fewer calories they eat, the better off they are. This doesn't work for everyone, especially for people who tend to get tired in the afternoon, feel dizzy or weak in the midmorning, and feel better after they eat.

Eating needs to be placed in context. Just as a calorie is not a calorie is not a calorie, the same applies to the timing of when you eat.

For people to benefit from breakfast, it's usually a good idea to have some protein during their breakfast. Studies show that people who do not eat breakfast end up eating more during the rest of the day to make up for it.

On the other end of the spectrum, intermittent fasting, which is a tradition in many cultures, has been shown to be of equal benefit, for those who are ready for it, in terms of losing weight. It helps to bring down blood lipid parameters. Additionally, it has been shown to protect and to help the healing of brain cells.[39,40,41,42]

For diabetics who can tolerate it, two larger meals daily are more effective than six smaller ones to control sugar levels, as well as weight. In one study, those who ate two meals a day, breakfast and lunch, also had lower liver fat content and increased insulin sensitivity than those who ate the same amount of calories spread over the course of the day.[43]

You might have noticed that I said not to skip meals, but also that intermittent fasting is OK if you are ready for it.[44] People who read medical research on a regular basis are not surprised to see studies in well-known scientific journals coming to different conclusions. It's a normal part of the growth curve of science.

For those with low blood sugar issues not skipping meals is helpful, since eating at regular times can stabilize fluctuating blood sugar levels. Including protein with these meals is important, as it also helps to maintain more stable sugar levels.

It's another example of the need for you to investigate and to come to your own conclusions, about what is best for your body.

Not all physicians will view the results of research in the same ways. Some doctors might minimize particular findings, while others might tout their importance and suggest your course of care based on them.

When Einstein published his first work on the theory of relativity, it was met with indifference in a number of scientific circles. He won a Nobel Prize later, but it was given to him for his discovery of the photoelectric effect, not for his world-changing theory of relativity. That theory was not seen as having the importance then that it does now.

I once read a biography of Einstein that mentioned how he had applied to several high schools to be a math teacher. He attached his article on the theory of relativity to his résumé but was turned down several times, never getting the job![45]

If we think of our body as a vehicle having varying degrees of health, like a car, it's easy to see how important it is for everything to work well. You can change the transmission, the oil, and even the engine, but it's not enough for any car to drive well.

You also need air in those tires!

What You Can Do Now

- Chew 10 to 30 times before swallowing to lose weight; that helps to kill bugs and improves your digestion.
- Drinking 16 ounces of water half an hour before meals will put a nice dent in your appetite levels. Add fiber, or eat soup, to supercharge the effect.
- Not every calorie is equal in its effect on your weight or on sugar levels in the future. If you are going to eat

emotionally, develop the habit of eating comfort food that has a fairly low glycemic load but still satisfies you.

- To help lower your blood sugar levels after a meal, don't sit for long periods of time throughout the day. After every 20 minutes of sitting, walk around for just two minutes to make a difference in your post-meal blood sugar levels, as well as to lower your insulin levels.[46]

- To fast or not to fast . . . it's an individual decision that works for some, while others may not have a body ready to handle it, especially if they have low blood sugar issues.

- What you eat, beyond counting calories, matters when trying to lose weight. Consider eating less refined food and more vegetables and protein sources. Don't eat high-fat junk meals when stressed; they cause weight gain.

- Go beyond the glycemic index and look at the glycemic load of foods. That's the more important index in determining what is better to eat while losing weight.

- Raw organic potato starch is one type of resistant starch. It can be found on the Internet or in health food stores. It works best raw. Mix it in lukewarm soup or water.

- If you don't digest proteins well, consider adding a nutritional supplement such as betaine hydrochloric acid. If you have low acid levels in your stomach, apart from not helping the body to digest and absorb nutrients well, it will diminish your body's ability to kill parasites and bugs from the food.

[28]

Gonna Keep Pumping Air in That Tire?

IF YOU REALIZED that one of your tires had low air pressure, would you put air into it?

Of course. But what if you were told that you had to pump air into your tires every day, probably for the rest your life, and that it was possible that, over time, you'd have to pump more and more air into them each day?

You would likely start questioning why and what to do about it. However, many people are told something similar in clinics every day throughout the country as they are handed prescriptions for medication. They are informed that these medications are for long-term or even lifetime use. Many patients accept the instructions without much questioning.

Question them!

Let's view the tire as an illness or a set of symptoms. You keep taking medicine for it every day, sometimes twice a day, but it doesn't improve on its own. It gets worse if you stop taking the medication, like having low air pressure in your tires every morning.

What does that tell you about simply continuing to take that approach, if you really want to get to the root of the problem?

Eighty percent of the time, when an average patient in this country goes to a doctor, he or she is prescribed drug therapy.[1] That's an awfully high number.

Think about it. Do we need prescription drugs for 80 percent of our problems? Remember when I mentioned earlier that up to 50 percent of antibiotic prescriptions were thought to be unnecessary? This was revealed in research from the *New England Journal of Medicine*.[2]

More than four billion prescriptions were written last year, and that number is rising. I noted that almost half of all Americans are on at least one prescription drug.

I'm a strong advocate for correct use of prescription drugs. In fact, I'm glad that we have them and look forward to new ones that will help when nothing else will. A patient and his prescribing doctor should carefully go over what's really needed and what can be put aside, or consider undergoing a trial therapeutic withdrawal if appropriate.

When it comes to overprescription issues, my thoughts go to application and context. If the only thing in your toolbox were a hammer, what do you think would happen every time you had to fix something in the house?

You'd likely try to use it for almost everything you could! That's what has been done with many prescriptions. They have been used too much, when other approaches would have been more appropriate.

My sense is that we serve the needs of a patient best by clinically exploring what can be done to support and help the rest of the body and its processes to respond best, whatever that person's condition or disease might be. We do this by looking for connections in the way the entire body functions.

At a fundamental level, long-term health is about interrelationships, about connections, associations, processes that help other parts of the body to heal, or that make it harder to recover, as we have seen. When some parts don't work well, other parts might have to compensate. I mentioned that it's like four people lifting a heavy piece of furniture when one of them is weak. The three others will feel the added stress of having to take up the slack.

A Quick Review

Let's briefly go over some of the topics we have been discussing:

We've talked a bit about your body being like a garden; that your health works just like a garden. We grow into good health, or experience bad health, similar to the dynamics of a garden.

We also touched on the topic of tightly knit global economic and social patterns that are a consequence of modern science and communication technology. I said that they, in turn, were a reflection of an age-old natural tradition used by older societies that could teach us more deeply how to heal our bodies.

No System Stands Alone

We also explored viewing the body as a whole, with body systems and organs that have strong and immediate effects on each other, and not as largely unrelated body parts to be medicated, or even treated with natural organic supplements. Later, we'll touch on other important connections, or aspects of your health, that go beyond the physical.

I am going to build up to that by placing our attention on your body's immune system and its relationship to you. For purposes of grouping them together, I refer to our body as having 12 systems. In reality, they are all connected and dependent on each other.

The immune system is commonly thought of as a separate system, but keep in mind that it depends on other systems to work well. No system in the body works like an island or stands alone. In this context, all systems work as a part of the immune system.

For example, you need your stomach to work well to create stomach acids that destroy parasites and bacteria that you ingest with food.

Your intestines destroy pathogenic microbes, while your liver is needed for detoxification and enzyme production. Your spleen synthesizes antibodies, while the nerves of your nervous system interact with immune cells in your gut.

Your lungs and bones also form part of your immune system. Your lungs produce their own defensive strategies against microbes; meanwhile, the long bones in your body create white blood cells to fight pathogens.

It's clear that you can't have an optimal immune response without other systems in the body working well and together. Even vitamins and trace minerals contribute to prevent problems that might arise from the effects of free radicals, by forming the basis of antioxidants.

Simply observing how seemingly unrelated parts and systems of our body are so closely interconnected can have a big impact on our health challenges. We need to go beyond our usual frame of thinking to look for underlying patterns that are affecting our health. Through information, questions, answers, and interchange, you can begin to see your health differently.

And make a change.

What You Can Do Now

- Beyond the concerns for side effects and drug–drug interactions, which we covered in more detail in the first chapter, there are three questions to ask yourself every time you are told that you need a prescription: What would likely happen if I don't take it? What is this drug trying to do that my body is not doing on its own? What natural support can I offer my body so that it can do more of what it needs to do on its own?

[29]

On Healing and Rainbows

IT TAKES A lot of energy and effort for a body to recuperate and to heal from most chronic health issues. The process of healing places a demand on our constitution.

Many patients don't realize that it can take a long time for their body to make fundamental changes after many years of depleting their health and recuperative reserves. Some look only for a quick change for their symptoms and might drop out of care before giving their body a chance to finally start healing at deeper levels.

Consistency and discipline to follow a well-planned program designed by any doctor or clinician is a cornerstone for long-term success. For some patients, that means a shift in viewpoint from simply wanting to continue to fill up their proverbial flat tires to exploring what it means to find and help to heal the underlying issues.

Everyone's different; clinical cookie-cutter approaches carry a lot of limitations. In my experience, what works best is that, as the conditions of my patients begin to improve, and as the cells and tissues of their bodies heal more and their healing forces express better health, they usually see them typically move from an initial program to a long-term plan to reach progressively higher levels of improvement.

Through periodic examinations and the monitoring of improvements, we can best determine next clinical steps, which in the course of care might include nutritional support based on individual body indicators, blood testing, imaging, and adjunctive therapies.

Initial Healing Responses

On the topic of varying patient responses to treatment, there's something that I see from time to time, and it's not just me but also a number of doctors who work with natural healing approaches. The body might sometimes go through what is known as *healing reactions,* or retracing, similar to what is known as a *Herxheimer* reaction.

It is named after a German dermatologist who more than 80 years ago observed that at times there was a pattern of response by the body to healing. Although the name of this reaction has been classically used to describe the body's inflammatory short-term reaction to the introduction of certain antibiotic medicines in some diseases, it's also commonly used to describe symptoms that patients might experience as they go through their healing cycle.

These are temporary, and usually pass pretty quickly; most people don't have them. For those who do, some might experience signs of inflammation, some might experience headaches, and others might feel some weakness or fatigue.

If your body is killing bugs or detoxifying more quickly than its detoxification and elimination capacity can handle, you may have some short-term symptoms.

Remember the research regarding supervised water fasting therapy and how it lowered high blood pressure? Every person in that study was informed that as their body began to detoxify, they would potentially experience similar reactions.

I tell patients at the beginning of their treatment that they might experience this type of reaction, to prepare them for any potential symptoms. They can then call us if that is the case. We can help. Sometimes it's as simple as helping to slow down the body's rate of detoxification and healing to a more comfortable pace.

Everyone responds differently, even if they come in with the same symptoms and are placed on the same treatment program. It's what makes this an interesting challenge for the clinician. Everyone's different, everyone has had different life experiences, and their bodies respond differently. We are, fortunately, unique.

We discussed that the human body is a complex, open-ended system. It changes as it interacts with its environment, including its internal environment.

Genetic Nutrition

A good example of this interdependence lies in the field of epigenetics. It is the study of how genes change the way they work due to environmental responses, without changing their coding. Nutrition might go a long way in helping to influence how genes express themselves. If you are interested in nutrition for good gene expression, as a baseline, it's particularly good to include B vitamins, curcumin, resveratrol, and sufficient sources of organic iron.

There is an interesting field in nutrition called *nutrigenomics*, which studies the individual interactions between nutrition and how an individual will respond based on his or her genes—how genes express themselves in response to the nutrients eaten.[1] Foods that would be most helpful according to the genetic profile of an individual are emphasized.

Researchers have shown that how you take care of your nutrition, especially when exposed to stress prior to childbirth, can affect at least two more generations. It could lead to a grandchild having a greater incidence of metabolic diseases such as diabetes or metabolic syndrome, even though he or she might not be overweight.[2,3,4,5,6,7,8,9]

The effect is not just from the mother's care but also influenced by how well the father takes care of himself.[10]

Our body has a fascinating and complex internal environment. We have approximately 37 trillion cells in our body, each one performing approximately 100,000 biochemical processes per second. And that's not counting the bacteria, viruses, and other bugs that live inside each of us—there are many more trillions of bacteria and viruses in our body.[11]

No doctor can monitor all bodily functions. It's why I am not only happy when patients tell me that they are experiencing positive changes; I am also a little relieved.

My intent and expectation is for everyone to get better. I am sure that all treating physicians in every discipline work hard toward that end. I know the body has an amazing capacity to heal itself when the conditions are right. I've seen and lived it.

At the same time, however, I recognize that it's the body that does the healing, and not the doctor.

Healing Is an Individual Experience

For me, the clinician does what he or she can, but ultimately, healing takes place as the result of the effects on our bodies of that life force that flows through each one of us. I believe that healing comes from this life force that gives structure, order, and purpose to the universe.

Perhaps a good analogy is to look at health and healing as a universal garden of life and each one of us as a small but important patch in it.

All that we doctors can really take credit for is listening, observing, and providing the patient with what we think will help make the best clinical changes, in accordance with how the patient's body, a reflection of nature, works. On the patient's part, patience and a measure of discipline are needed. But we have to wait to see how the healing system will respond. Everyone's different.

Will it respond quickly or slowly? Will it respond in a way that leads to deep healing, or might there just be some superficial changes? If the body is not healing, are there deeper issues that need to be looked at, perhaps beyond clinical reach?

That's why one of the first things I tell patients is that if I don't see results after a reasonable period of time, after I have tried what I think should work well, I'll refer them to someone who I think might help better, and we can work as a team as needed.

Sometimes, based on the initial examination or screening test results from lab work or imaging studies, I refer them to another doctor right away. The important thing is for each patient to find a doctor who best suits his or her health needs. There are great doctors in every healing art.

Doctors of all branches of health, whether working with drugs or only through natural means, are part of a global healing community, even if they're not aware of it. Ideally, we would work side by side, making sure the patients were under the care of the clinicians best suited for them, while connecting and communicating, sharing and learning, from one another.

Similar to today's deep economic and communication ties with distant and foreign cultures, physicians would reach out and establish connections with other physicians who followed different healing traditions.

Earlier, I touched on the obvious importance of biodiversity for our planet's health. It speaks of the need for keeping alive the many different types of plants and animals, because they all contribute in some way. That also applies at a clinical level, among doctors and healers.

We can extend that concept of biodiversity by including a wide range of diverse clinical approaches from all fields of health, and embracing divergent and seemingly competing or contradictory clinical perspectives from different cultures.

The end result is a healthier ecosystem within the body of each patient.

To illustrate that, let's use the rainbow as an example, while posing a question: for you, which is the most important color in the rainbow?

The Colors of Diversity

We usually like some colors more than others, true, but most of us would agree that all are equally important, or it simply wouldn't be a rainbow. That's how health care can be seen. Every color in the rainbow of health, every clinical approach, whether mainstream or alternative, is valid and useful. Everything has its place and purpose.

The clinician who experiences the deepest results is the one who is willing to work, in effect, with all the colors available in the healing spectrum. That means reaching out to those in other disciplines of health who have a deeper knowledge about a particular color, or aspect, of their patient's health—embracing clinical diversity.

The colors of the rainbow touch one another; they're not separated. Why should the way we treat our body or the way doctors view working with those in other fields be different? What would happen if the connectivity and interaction dynamics that I have given examples of among body systems and organs and nature were applied by the worldwide community of doctors?

It would give patients their best chance of healing, and along the way transform the way people think and experience their health, with a more integrated perspective.

In putting all of our efforts into regaining health, a question arises that is often overlooked, similar to the metaphor of continuing to inflate the flat tires in our health without questioning where the leaks are.

Someone once said that man spends the first part of his life using his health to accumulate wealth and spends the second part of his life spending his wealth to accumulate health.

We rarely put attention on the why of being healthy, since it seems so obvious. Yet, other than helping us to feel good and allowing us to function better, what, then, is the purpose of health?

What You Can Do Now

- Our bodies do not work in a linear way; neither does our healing. When you start a clinical program to help to improve the function of your body, if you don't feel well, check with the clinician to see if you are having a healing reaction.
- Having an open mind and being willing to experiment within the realm of clinical reason with other approaches to healing is one of the biggest gifts that physicians can offer their patients.
- It's a big, wide world of clinical rainbows. Why limit standard health care approaches to just a couple of rays of color?

[30]

Your Body Is Your Garden

AFTER A MARRIAGE of more than 30 years, her husband passed away due to pancreatic cancer. Toward the end, while lying in his hospital bed, he kept telling her how grateful he was to have had her and their children in his life, that he considered himself fortunate. He kept repeating to always keep an open heart for life's blessings.

As he approached the end of his life, their relationship had drastically changed, shifting from one of conflict to one of compassion and grace.

However, that probably would not have happened without his terminal illness.

In fact, he changed so much during it. He became more loving, more compassionate, and more grateful for the gifts in his life.

As his condition worsened, he became more graceful and loving.

He wasn't like that before while he was in good health. His experience with cancer helped to heal these other, nonphysical aspects. He used to be a pretty tough guy, and he had a strong personality. Self-reliant, strong and judgmental, he expected and demanded strength and self-reliance from others.

When he became ill, he lost that physical strength and had to accept the help of those around him, mostly his family members. These acts of kindness eventually awoke a greater compassion in him toward others.

He realized that his survival depended on the love and compassion that his family freely and lovingly gave him, over and over again. He began to gracefully accept the sacrifices that they made for him, their acts of love helping his hardened heart to open. In his last days, he was filled with immense gratitude, love, and expressions of affection.

Through this trying and life-ending experience, he became a softer, more thoughtful and considerate man. The irony is that his pancreatic cancer, this terrible illness, was at the same time a healing salve for his mental and emotional wounds.

Sometimes illness teaches us more than the experience of good health ever can. Whatever our level of health is, there is usually a golden nugget of wisdom associated with it that can help us take a better step forward in our life if we reflect on and absorb its lessons.

Health and illness, which most people think of as polar opposites, are more deeply intertwined than we are commonly aware of. A deeper understanding of ourselves, our essence, can make a big difference in our lives as well as in the lives of those we touch.

So far, we've focused on these interconnected systems of health primarily as biological processes. However, we've also explored a number of emotional and mental components regarding food choices, and discussed how emotions can affect the body, such as chronic lower back pain.

If health can be likened to a wheel, with our identity, who we are, at its axis, perhaps we could gain a more complete understanding of what more fully defines health if we imagine a wheel with four spokes running from the axis to the rim. Each spoke would represent our physical, emotional, mental, and spiritual dynamics. The rim would be considered our daily life.

The axis would represent who we, in essence, are. Our nervous system, comprised of our brain, spinal cord and nerves, expresses these four dynamics, the spokes of the wheel of health, through our body. The state of our health is a reflection of the interplay among these four important aspects.

To find out more about the roles that they play in health and healing, let's go back a few thousand years to learn from the wisdom expressed in ancient civilizations.

We will visit with the Greeks and the Romans shortly, but first let me ask: Where does the word *health* come from?

It comes from an old Saxon word meaning "whole." In its root definition, *health* means wholeness, or being whole. Knowing more about what that means can make a significant difference in our health challenges.

Let's explore that.

What You Can Do Now

- Consider keeping a journal where you explore what a deeper aspect of you is trying to tell you through an illness. Look to see what secondary gains, positive and negative, an illness or condition has brought to your life.
- Is it distracting you from facing other things? How it is changing the way you see and feel about yourself? How has it changed the ways that others are treating you? Has it changed the level of love and compassion toward yourself or others?
- If you assumed, just for the purposes of this journal, that your condition had something to teach you, begin to write what that could be, and see where this

process takes you. If your condition has created a situation in which you're not facing some uncomfortable issues, write about those as well.

[31]

The Essential You: Deeper Meanings to Illness

THE ANCIENT GREEKS believed that when you were ill, it was because you had lost harmony with yourself and with life. Symptoms were viewed as a loss of harmony and balance.

This viewpoint about the relationship between a person's balance, internal harmony, and harmony with life was shared by a number of ancient healing cultures, including Native Americans, Romans, and shamanistic societies throughout the world.

Restoring health, then, was seen as restoring harmony and integrity within oneself and with life—a mirror of one's internal state.

That's quite different from the modern health care typically received. When you see your doctors, you tell them what's going on, they might do some testing, and then you are usually given prescriptions in an attempt to get you back to where you were before you became ill.

There is nothing inherently wrong with that approach. It's just that what we are discussing here involves additional parameters, including those of mind and spirit.

Most people believe that all aspects of life have a purpose, whatever you might believe that purpose or belief system to be. Since illness and disease are part of life, if we accept the premise that all of life has a purpose or meaning, then what is the purpose of illness, of disease?

This is simply an exploration, so there are no hard and fast answers that anyone can give you, as we discussed earlier about philosophy.

Philosophy cannot be proved. There are things you choose to believe and act upon that can bring you more fulfilling life experiences. They can lead you to a deeper and more integrated sense of who you are and of your relationship with your purpose in life.

Health and Wholeness

Those who believe that all of life's experiences have something to teach us are aligned with the viewpoint of many ancient cultures and traditions that believed that the central part of us, who we really are, came into this life with a purpose, with goals.

In other words, they believed that we are here for a reason.

They believed that good health is a reflection of this central aspect of ourselves, the essence of who we are beyond biology, or that which Swiss psychologist Carl Jung called the "Self." When a person is not aligned with her highest purpose, illness and disease arose as a signal and as a consequence. It served as an indicator that she has lost her highest perspective.

Instead of only treating symptoms or conditions, they would explore ill health as an indicator of deeper life meanings.

Let's travel a few thousand miles and a couple of thousand years back in time to observe an example of this. The Romans used to have healing temples throughout their empire. A requisite to enter one of these temples and to receive healing was for the person to come to terms with his illness, to reconcile himself, since it was believed that without doing so, there could be no true healing.[1]

Just what does "coming to terms" mean? Is that reconciliation? Carl Jung spoke of health and healing as a process of the unconscious becoming conscious. He called that process "individuation," which involves the integration of the conscious mind, or ego, and the unconscious, or central aspect of the person: the Self.

He believed that the nature of this internal, central Self was a yearning for wholeness, equivalent to the yearning for God. He spoke of illness and disease as being the crucible where this transformation took place, and that only in this Self could healing take place and the person be made whole.[2]

These concepts about health and wholeness have a bearing on our symptoms and our biological functions, our health. But they can also go much deeper and have a bigger impact on our lives. It's a deeper viewpoint of health that is important for our healing, in the most profound sense of the word.

For many, it forms a key point to attaining health. It does not discount clinical treatment for these symptoms and illnesses; they should not be ignored. We've made wonderful technological advances in the science of healing and should take advantage of them whenever possible.

One of the topics we've been exploring is that symptoms and diseases can be the consequences, or expressions, of deeper dysfunctional patterns of cells and tissues in our body.

Instances might arise that allow us to discover that the root causes of our illnesses go beyond physical dysfunction. An illness might be a symptom, a consequence, of a loss of balance by the ancient definition of health at deeper levels: a loss of wholeness.

It could be related to a loss, or dysfunction, between a person and the balance and harmony of nature and its laws. On that same note, it's interesting to see how wholeness-based approaches to health has been treated in many spiritual works across continents and millennia.

Let's look at some examples.

- In the ancient Indian *ayurvedic* healing system, the relationship between the patient and nature is central. The practitioner's intent is to help the patient balance her physical, emotional, and spiritual aspects. In this system, yoga is used as a tool to bring balance to these three aspects.

- In the New Testament, more than once, when Jesus is telling someone that he or she has been healed, he uses the phrase "made whole."
- In traditional Chinese medicine, all aspects of a person's health are used for diagnosis—not just the physical and nutritional, but also the emotional, mental, and spiritual aspects. The intent is to return to a balance of the energies flowing through the patient.

These examples might remind you of similarities with the philosophy of chiropractic that I detailed earlier. All of these approaches, from different eras, countries, and even religions, share a viewpoint on who we essentially are: spiritual beings in deep resonance with the rhythms of life.

So does this mean that illness and disease were viewed as a message that something was wrong with the spiritual aspect of a person?

I don't see it in terms of right or wrong. I think more along the lines of illness being an indicator that there has been a loss of connection, a loss of a fuller expression with our inner harmony or with the laws of nature.

I view illness as an invitation to explore the central aspects of ourselves more deeply—in other words, an opportunity for lessons to be learned. At least, that's my understanding: that the loss of health can cause us to tune in at deeper levels, a painful opportunity for connection, rebalancing, and growth.

It does not mean that every time someone is sick, he needs to look for a deeper connection with life and within himself. Many times this loss of balance or harmony can take place at a simple level.

Here's an example. How many times did you eat something that your body simply didn't agree with? Well, the solution might be simple—stop eating it!

Sometimes healing can be as easy as getting the right information about possible nutritional deficiencies or therapeutic approaches that work for us at that moment. Other times, it might be as simple as putting on a pair of your favorite sneakers and going out for a brisk walk.

At a biological level, your body is like a laboratory. Test to see what works well for it and what does not. Everyone is unique and might respond differently. The passing of time will also bring changes in how your body works and responds to foods and therapies that once worked well.

We don't have to make a big deal of it every time we feel bad. Sometimes it's as simple as saying no to one type of food and yes to another that's better for you. Or, you might reflect on a problem that isn't clearing up and get an intuitive sense that it is time to change doctors. Help can come indirectly, in many ways.

It's a relief not to have to think that every little health problem has to be overly complicated. It's nice to know that there can be simple solutions at times; in fact, that's the way it is a lot of the time.

There are instances when there is no need to look for deeper symbolism. Sometimes a simple stomachache is just a simple stomachache, like many people have after eating a heavy late-night meal.

Healing Beyond the Body

There also might be times when a condition or an illness is not being cured and goes beyond the reach of the usual clinical approaches.

These might be the times when turning to whatever instruments of introspection and insight you have would be useful. Establishing contact with the deeper aspect of yourself and your relationship with the harmony and laws of nature not only can lead to better health but, if the condition is serious enough, could perhaps save your life.

The challenge for many people is determining where to start when a problem doesn't go away, no matter how many doctors they've seen or cures they've tried.

If you are among those who believe that life and every experience in it has a reason, a purpose, a structure, then when every appropriate clinical approach has been tried, it might be time to consider using whatever emotional, mental, and spiritual tools you have available in your life's toolbox to seek answers that might lie beyond strictly physical or biochemical dynamics.

It could be an approach at whatever level felt right for you to explore; this is a personal experience and every person is different.

You need to find your own answers, sometimes with the help of those around you.

Patients have asked me what I mean by a life toolbox. It's about choosing what instruments, or life tools, can help you. Everyone has to find what they feel works best for them. I can only give you suggestions.

For example, you could consult with a priest or a minister of a religion you feel comfortable with. Sometimes traveling to new lands and experiencing how others approach life differently can give us needed insights as well. Mark Twain said that travel kills ignorance. I've lived in five countries and moved around a lot since I was born, a process that has taught me a lot about myself. Others might not need to travel or live abroad for their experiences.

A person could undergo therapy with a professional to explore what might be out of line with her sense of internal peace and harmony. Sometimes just talking to a close friend who listens well really helps. Each approach can be different, a custom fit.

Bodywork, which can include chiropractic, massage, yoga, t'ai chi, Rolfing, or acupuncture, among other modalities, can be helpful. There is an old saying, "The issues are in the tissues." There are many instances where the right type of bodywork helped an individual to become more aware of—and to ultimately release—deep chronic patterns.

Some other tools that can help a person to consciously align with this balance and harmony include meditating, keeping a diary of life events, writing down dreams, and doing spiritual contemplative exercises.

Something that works quite well to help you to view your life and its gifts in context, and to help you to keep an open heart through difficult times, is to keep a gratitude journal. Just write down every day, no matter how tough the day was, at least a few things that you were grateful for. Then make sure to read through your gratitude journal from time to time.

There are many other tools, of course, some of which you can create yourself. It is important for a person to find the precise approach that helps open his or her heart to a greater understanding.

Perhaps all of our deepest healings come from our hearts.

Many wonder if their disease will go away if they look deeper within themselves. Each person is different, and his or her life experiences, including those related to health and healing, will be different. Healing can come in different ways. It might not always be expressed physically.

Ancient healers and philosophers taught that physical healing has a much better chance of taking place once a person's core beliefs and central purpose in life are reintegrated into his daily actions. How that plays out in the life of any particular person is something we cannot predict.

What is certain is that an important shift must take place at a deeper level that consciously aligns us with our essential self and purpose.

That, by itself, is healing.

What You Can Do Now

- If you are willing, assume for the purpose of this exercise that an illness or condition that you have not been able to resolve for a long time has a message for you, as painful or joyful as it may be.

- Assume that it concerns what you came here to do in your life, at the deepest level, beyond the roles that you have been playing in society and with family and friends. Explore that sense of who you are at the deepest level and what you may not have been fully expressing about yourself. Write it down and perhaps talk with close friends and with people you trust to get a sense for how they see you either stuck or evolving within this process.

- Perhaps you have already made wonderful strides through it, and what is left to do is to simply allow time for thetissues of your body, if possible within the limitations of time and matter, to heal as best as they can.

- Perhaps your condition is a profound invitation to inquire within.

[32]

Help for Deep Healing: Life's Toolbox

IF YOU HAVE a disease or a problem that won't go away, no matter what you have tried, it might be time to look more deeply for ways to facilitate healing the inner aspects of your life. Your body might be acting as a mirror to call attention to an important part of you that needs healing.

If so, ask yourself what your condition might be revealing about you. There are a number of other things you can do that will help you to look inside more closely, to recognize patterns that need attention.

I don't have the final word, or even close to a complete one, but a lot of times it helps to start with something that can be as simple as physical exercise, if the circumstances permit. It gets your energy flowing and has beneficial effects on the brain and the body.

When you do exercise, especially higher-intensity exercise, a substance known as *brain-derived neurotrophic factor* is produced. It helps a number of nerve cells to regenerate. It also helps other nerve cells to create better connections with each other and to survive. It helps a part of the brain involved with memory, the hippocampus, to grow, even in senior citizens; and this substance also helps with long-term memory, learning, and reasoning.[1,2,3]

You can pray, meditate, or do spiritual contemplative exercises. Carl Jung spoke about the use of active imagination when doing contemplative exercises, suggesting that you enter into a conscious internal dialogue with yourself about your dreams.

It's best to find something that works for you, since everyone is different and has different needs.

If you are a Christian, for example, perhaps repeating the Lord's Prayer or another devotional prayer would be helpful. If you practice or are open to the healing tools of an Eastern faith, such as Hinduism, there are rituals, ceremonies, and meditations that involve repeating a single word, "Om," that could be helpful. Zen meditation practices have been commonly used for over a thousand years. People in many countries, even from different religions, have benefited from them.

Some people meditate in a secular way, as in Transcendental Meditation.[4] Some chant or sing a variety of words, such as "HU," an ancient name for God, to develop a stronger relationship with the Spirit.[5] I sing "HU" daily. Others simply repeat a word or a number over and over to enter into a deeper contemplative stillness.

I remember as a kid reading a lot of *National Geographic* magazines that my parents had lying around the house. I read with curiosity and wonder about dances and drum circles from all over the world in which people attempted to contact their deeper aspects. Whirling dervishes, for example, do this through dancing and praying.

Working on a physical level, even for issues that involve mental, emotional, or spiritual dynamics—and for me they are all connected—is important. As the mind affects the body, so does the body affect the mind and the psyche.

When you breathe slowly, at approximately five in-and-out breaths a minute if you can, you help to activate the part of your nervous system that relaxes you and aids in healing and regeneration.[6,7,8,9,10] One way you can do this is by counting to two while breathing in, then pause slightly and breathe out while counting to four. You can substitute the words *joy* or *peace* for the numbers while you do it. If six seconds is too long, try counting to one on the in-breath and to two on the out-breath.

Other tools you can use at home involve simple devices that help you to change the way your heart beats, and improve your health, by putting attention on positive emotions while you breathe. You can find more information at HeartMath (http://heartmath.com). These tools that change how the body functions by working with the breath and emotions can also help people with high blood pressure whether or not they are taking medications, according to research.[11]

The interconnectedness within our body extends to all parts of us; the web that we weave creates oscillations that run through the threads of our physical, emotional, mental, and spiritual selves.

We have a wonderful set of life tools at our disposal within us, waiting to be explored and used for our happiness and well-being. The more closely we align with and engage that deeper part of us, the easier it is to access inner sources of wisdom, such as our intuition, as well as healing.

Dreams as a Health Tool

Another way of discovering more about yourself in a way that can make a meaningful impact on your health is through the study of your dreams.

The significance of dreams to the inner journey of humans, and their healing forces, has been written in the pages of wise and ancient spiritual traditions throughout the globe.

I've already mentioned the Romans and their healing temples. Being able to enter a temple for healing was a selective process. To be invited in, you had to receive a dream invitation. You were questioned about your dreams to see if you were an acceptable candidate. Once you went through the process and were finally admitted to the temple, you could spend days there in the hope that a healing dream would cure you.[12]

There was a famous physician by the name of Claudius Galen whose works left a lasting impression on Western medicine. Galen served as the physician for emperors and many Roman senators. Among his many discoveries was that the nervous system, through the nerves in our body, controls the contraction of our muscles.

Galen believed that doctors should be philosophers as well as healers, combining philosophy with medical practice. His unique approach to medicine was, at its roots, very open to trying new things and not being rigid in one school or style of medical practice.[13]

He is an example of someone who applied new clinical approaches to health care, who looked at things differently and demonstrated how the old can teach the new, the new being willing.

In breaking "new" ground 2,000 years ago, Galen became the preeminent doctor in the history of Western medicine. Although his science and methods are out of date, the freshness and vitality of his thinking, his openness to new ideas, and his impact made him an extraordinary presence in the annals of medical history.

If he were alive today, he would probably press for changes in our health care system. He wasn't one to practice the way his predecessors did for the sake of continuity.

For example, one way that Galen diagnosed patients was by asking them about their dreams.[14] We've moved in a much different direction since Galen's time. The seduction of modern science and medicine, with its many necessary wonders, has also left many a doctor blind to what the eyes of ancient physicians saw as important to healing.

Galen became a physician because his father dreamed that his son should become one; this highlights the importance of dreams in these ancient societies. In modern times, we have lost this important connection. Modern society places little attention on dreams.

Following in the wisdom of ancient cultures, we can use dreams as a guide to our health problems.

If that is an area of interest to you, what can you do to help yourself if, like many others, you don't remember your dreams?

What You Can Do Now

- Breathing techniques as well as mindful attention to your heartbeat have been shown to be helpful with high blood pressure, even if you are on medication for that. They can also help to lower stress levels. The citations in this chapter on this topic will lead you to more information. Another resource is HeartMath (http://heartmath.com).

- If you can, exercise. If you can't . . . exercise. In some way. Even if it's just your mind.

- If nothing else, lie down and exercise the gift of imagination, as you give wings to your highest and most deeply held dreams.

- What's your favorite prayer or chant of solace? That's a spiritual remedy.

- Perhaps the best remedy of all: find more ways of serving others.

[33]

Dreaming Your Way to Better Health

DREAMS ARE A reflection of our inner world, and since each one of us is traveling on our own individual journey, their meanings and significance will be unique to us. My sense is that it's up to every one of us, as part of our journey, to figure out their meanings.

When I was young and my parents took me to the movies, my mother would distract me when the couple on the screen started to kiss. It took me a long time to figure out what she was doing. She thought I was too young to see it!

Dreams are similar to this. It can take a while to figure out what they mean—and they always mean something, at some level.

One reason they can appear to be confusing is because the contents of our subconscious, our inner world, without the context of symbolism could be distressing to the conscious mind.

It helps to write your dreams in a diary and later match them to what has been going on in your life. It might give you insights into the symbolism and the meaning of your dreams. It can also help illuminate the internal dynamics of persistent health issues.

Dreams are more than just symbols, but it's a good start. Often, it's as if your body is trying to send you a message about your health, but you have to decrypt it first to understand its meaning.

When you wake up, briefly write down whatever dreams you remember. Our mind has a sensor that distorts our dream images, so the impact of dreams on our waking life is lessened. Don't worry if they don't make sense initially. Just briefly write down the highlights of what you do remember.

If you have difficulty remembering your dreams, just before you go to sleep, repeat to yourself softly a few times that you will remember your dreams upon awakening, and have a notepad and pen at your bedside. Then go to sleep, and when you wake up, before opening your eyes, spend a moment or two playing back your dreams. With practice, this has helped many people to remember their dreams.

But even if you remember your dreams, how do you figure out what they mean, and how can they help you with your health issues?

The Benefit of Reviewing Dreams

One thing you can do is to go back and review your dreams once or twice a month and compare them with what has been going on in your life during that period. Over time, you will see patterns. You might see repeating images that reflect your personal symbols—doorways into the meaning of your inner worlds. Everyone's dream symbols, like their life experiences, are unique, and it might take time to develop a deeper understanding of what yours mean to you.

You can also check to see if there is a connection between your dreams and an illness. Sometimes it might not be direct. For example, when I do something that isn't healthy for my body, I often dream that something unpleasant is happening to me, even though it seems unrelated to what is going on in my physical life. You can learn to keep an eye out for these types of clues to find your symbols.

I've noticed that in my dreams, a green car has often been symbolic of my physical body—my physical vehicle. I notice the condition of the car, what's going on with it that might suggest problems or issues to come with my health.

Sometimes you get a sense when reviewing your dreams that you might need to move in a different direction with the type of treatment you are receiving or see a different doctor. That's why a dream diary can be so useful. You might not draw upon the wisdom of your dream that day, but later on, with the benefit of hindsight and in the context of your other dreams during that time, you can end up with good insights about your physical illness or other life problems.

Here's an example from my life. I was working on a project with a business professional for a few months. I had invested a lot of time and money in it but had a sense that his attention was on other business interests. I wasn't sure whether I should continue working with him.

I didn't know what to do. Then I had a dream experience that pointed the way for me. In it, he and I were in a house, and we were being attacked by archers shooting arrows at us. I knew that they wanted to invade the house and harm us. This person was with me in the house, but he was doing little to defend us. I was doing most of it on my own.

I woke up and reassessed the situation because I wanted to make sure that the dream was in line with other indicators. I took the dream into account in this case, but I always use my common sense when making decisions, to see what other information can be helpful. That dream alerted me to the need to make a change, which I did. A few weeks later, I found out that this partner was about to embark on a large and ambitious project, which would have left very little time for him to pay attention to the needs of our project.

I mentioned above that cars in my dreams seem to indicate that I should pay attention to something having to do with my body. A learning experience that I had about a car comes to mind, although in writing this I was embarrassed to share it. It had to do with a used car that I bought back when I was in school. I was practically broke and had to be careful about not just buying a car but also making sure that I wouldn't spend a lot of money on repairs until I graduated and started to work.

I saw a little brown car that I really liked. It seemed almost too good to be true—because it was. But I was young and inexperienced, and my judgment was led by my emotions. Shortly before buying the car, I dreamed that it was underwater. It was a short dream, and I dismissed it and went ahead and excitedly bought the car.

You might have already guessed how this story turned out. It was a terrible purchase! I had that little brown car for about four years because I couldn't afford another one, but in those four years the repair costs were higher than what I paid for the car. I took it to the garage so often that I became friends with the mechanic and his wife, who helped run the small garage.

One day I told the mechanic about the dream while shaking my head at yet another repair bill. This time the engine was beginning to sink on its support structure. The mechanic led me to the car and showed me some rusted bolts under the car's carpet, saying that he thought my dream was spot-on.

Whether for economic or health issues, really for anything that is important, we do have a wonderful inner resource to tap into and use as a guide to make better decisions—our dream world.

What You Can Do Now

- Write down five things you are grateful for when you get up each morning, changing them daily. Gratitude is a muscle that must be exercised.

- Also write down in your journal each morning what you remember from your dreams the night before. Review your dreams periodically, as well as your expressions of gratitude, for clues as to what direction to take next.

- If you don't remember what you dream, you can use the journal to write and later review events in your daily life that are significant to you, as well as how you feel about them. It can give you insights about your patterns of response to life experiences that you otherwise would not be aware of. Review it monthly.

[34]
The Reason Why

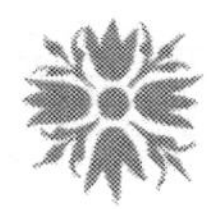

IN ANCIENT CULTURES, spiritual dreaming was an art, an important bridge between everyday life and one's inner worlds.

Working with dreams can give you deeper insights into your life. There are a number of books that can help on the subject of dreams.

Since you are different from everyone else, your interpretation of your dreams and the symbols in your inner life might be different from others'. Look for the books that can guide you in this individual, personalized direction. Seek books written by those who have experienced the significance of dreams at the deepest levels. They will probably be able to help you the most.[1,2,3]

Understanding your dream symbolism through dream journals and reviewing them over time can also help you to see patterns in your life. I write down my dreams every day in a journal because it helps me to better understand the relationship between my thoughts and how I am living my life. I review my journal every month. I also write down 15 affirmations daily, under the dream entry for that day, to help me center on what is important in my life. Affirmations are sentences that express how you want to be, or how you would like your life to be.

I have also found that daily contemplative exercises help me to understand and experience my dreams with more clarity and deeper meaning. Some dreams are not symbolic; they are direct, like the one about my car. Over time, with practice, you can make a better connection with your inner worlds through this resource.

We have been exploring health, illness, and disease as they relate to the central part of us, who we essentially are—what Carl Jung referred to as the Self. Here's another word for the Self: *Soul,* or inner essence. We have been exploring how our health status can reflect the balance, harmony, and inner fulfillment that each one of us is striving to attain.

What that fulfillment is, and how it manifests in our life, will be different for each of us, yet over the years I have seen a pattern as it relates to the improvement of the health of many patients.

Usually the initial phase of care involves patients' wanting to suppress painful or uncomfortable expressions of dysfunction in their body: symptoms. They put a lot of attention on that, which is natural and appropriate.

I rarely get patients who, coming in for the first time, either describe on the intake forms or express as their chief complaint an inability to do as much for their family as they would like to. Their attention and concern, appropriately enough, is to feel and to function better.

It's a priority for me to make this happen, to help to ease their pains. As they start feeling better, as their body begins to heal and they feel more energy and ease, many share with me, without my asking, that they are able to do more for their family and loved ones, and that they look forward to doing more for and with them.

They often bring out in our conversations, many times with their partner at their side, how their improved health allows them to help others more easily. Having a stronger and healthier body is often aligned with a natural desire to help others.

I've also witnessed how serious illnesses have brought forth greater levels of understanding and compassion in patients who, when physically healthy, had difficulties being present for others and expressing love.

The repetition of unhealthy patterns, at all levels, brings to many people frustration and pain for most of their lives, often affecting their health without their knowing it.

Perhaps life's greatest natural remedy, its natural prescription, consists of the applied wisdom that we can gain from the study of ancient cultures: simply observing how a garden flourishes, and immersing ourselves wholeheartedly in the complexities and opportunities that modern living brings to us.

Recently, a patient who over time had seen her health and vitality return, gratefully and lovingly shared how much more loving and giving she had become during this journey. It was a touching moment.

After she left, I leaned back in my chair and smiled. Looking out my office window, I rested my eyes on the yellow tulips and white gardenias in my small garden.

My gaze then shifted toward a grove of oak trees in the distance and to the swaying, windswept tips of tall, verdant pines that extended into the clear blue sky, each tree a dancing testament to the beauty and wonder of nature.

I thought of her and wondered to myself: perhaps those dancing green pine tips, like that patient, were doing what all of us were placed here to do, in sickness or in health.

To reach out and touch others through our highest purpose:

To love and to serve.

Notes

Chapter 2: Health Care: Beware the Hidden Risks

1. Lindsley CW. **The top prescription drugs of 2011 in the United States: Antipsychotics and antidepressants once again lead CNS therapeutics.** *ACS Chemical Neuroscience.* 2012;3(8):630.
2. **World Drug Report 2011.** United Nations Office on Drugs and Crime. http://www.unodc.org/documents/data-and-analysis/WDR2011/World_Drug_Report_2011_ebook.pdf.
3. **Drugs average 70 side effects.** UPI. May 24, 2011. http://www.upi.com/Health_News/2011/05/24/Drugs-average-70-side-effects/UPI-22001306295135/.
4. U.S. Food and Drug Administration. **Why Learn about Adverse Drug Reactions (ADR)?** http://www.fda.gov/Drugs/DevelopmentApprovalProcess/DevelopmentResources/DrugInteractionsLabeling/ucm114848.htm.
5. Lazarou J, Pomeranz BH, Corey PN. **Incidence of adverse drug reactions in hospitalized patients: A meta-analysis of prospective studies.** *Journal of the American Medical Association.* April 15, 1998;279:1200–1205.
6. Gu Q, Dillon C, Burt V. **Prescription drug use continues to increase: U.S. prescription drug data for 2007–2008.** Centers for Disease Control. September 2010. http://www.cdc.gov/nchs/data/databriefs/db42.htm.
7. Mansi I, et al. **Statins and New-Onset Diabetes Mellitus and Diabetic Complications: A Retrospective Cohort Study of US Healthy Adults.** *Journal of General Internal Medicine.* April 28, 2015.
8. Ibid.
9. Hopkins, AL. **Network pharmacology: The next paradigm in drug discovery.** *Nat Chem Bio.* November 2008;4(11):682–90.
10. Zhao S, Iyengar R. **Systems pharmacology: Network analysis to identify multiscale mechanisms of drug action.** *Annu Rev Pharmacol Toxicol.* 2012;52:505–21.
11. Hicks LA, Taylor TH Jr., Hunkler RJ. **U.S. outpatient antibiotic prescribing, 2010.** *N Engl J Med.* April 2013;368(15):1461–62.
12. Barnett ML, Linder JA. **Antibiotic prescribing to adults with sore throat in the United States, 1997–2010.** *JAMA Intern Med.* October 3, 2013;174(1):138–40.
13. Ibid.
14. Blaser M. **Antibiotic overuse: Stop the killing of beneficial bacteria.** *Nature.* August 24, 2011;476(7361):393–94.
15. Hviid A, Svanström H, Frisch M. **Inflammatory bowel disease: Antibiotic use and inflammatory bowel diseases in childhood.** *Gut.* 2011;60:149–54.
16. Mikkelsen KH, et al. **Use of Antibiotics and Risk of Type 2 Diabetes: A Population-Based Case-Control Study.** *J Clin Endocrinol Metab.* 2015 Aug 27:jc20152696. (Epub ahead of print.) PubMed PMID: 26312581.
17. **Antibiotic/antimicrobial resistance.** Centers for Disease Control and Prevention. http://www.cdc.gov/drugresistance/about.html. Updated August 6, 2014.
18. **Get smart for healthcare.** Centers for Disease Control and Prevention. http://www.cdc.gov/getsmart/healthcare. Updated May 28, 2014.
19. Teillant A. et al. **Potential burden of antibiotic resistance on surgery and cancer chemotherapy antibiotic prophylaxis in the USA: a literature review and modelling study.** *Lancet Infect Dis.* October 15, 2015.
20. Fitchett JR. **Antibiotics, copayments, and antimicrobial resistance: investment matters.** *The Lancet Infectious Diseases.* 15(10):1125–27.
21. Gupta S, et al. **Garlic: An Effective Functional Food to Combat the Growing Antimicrobial Resistance.** *Pertanika Journal of Tropical Agricultural Science.* 2015;38(2):271–78.
22. Ibid.
23. Tomas ME, et al. **Over-Diagnosis of Urinary Tract Infection and Under-Diagnosis of Sexually Transmitted Infection in Adult Women Presenting to an Emergency Department.** *J Clin Microbiol.* 2015;53(8):2686.
24. Kennedy P. **The Fat Drug.** *New York Times.* March 8, 2014. http://www.nytimes.com/2014/03/09/opinion/sunday/the-fat-drug.html?src=me&ref=general&_&_r=0.
25. Nobel YR, et al. **Metabolic and metagenomic outcomes from early-life pulsed antibiotic treatment.** *Nature Communications.* 2015;6:7486.

26. Kennedy P. **The Fat Drug.** *New York Times*. March 8, 2014. http://www.nytimes.com/2014/03/09/opinion/sunday/the-fat-drug.html?src=me&ref=general&_&_r=0.
27. Cox LM, et al. **Altering the intestinal microbiota during a critical developmental window has lasting metabolic consequences.** *Cell*. August 14, 2014;158(4):705–21.
28. **Therapeutic drug use.** Centers for Disease Control/National Center for Health Statistics. http://www.cdc.gov/nchs/fastats/drugs.htm. Updated May 14, 2014.
29. Meeker D, et al. **Nudging guideline-concordant antibiotic prescribing: A randomized clinical trial.** *JAMA Intern Med*. March 2014;174(3):425–31.
30. **Opioid painkiller prescribing: Where you live makes a difference.** Centers for Disease Control and Prevention: CDC VitalSigns. http://www.cdc.gov/vitalsigns/opioid-prescribing/index.html. Updated July 1, 2014.
31. Ibid.
32. **Vital signs: Overdoses of prescription opioid pain relievers and other drugs among women—United States, 1999–2010.** Centers for Disease Control and Prevention: Morbidity and Mortality Weekly Report (MMWR). 2013;62(26):537–42. http://www.cdc.gov/mmwr.
33. **Opioid painkiller prescribing: Where you live makes a difference.** Centers for Disease Control and Prevention: CDC VitalSigns. http://www.cdc.gov/vitalsigns/opioid-prescribing/index.html. Updated July 1, 2014.
34. Gooseens H, et al. **Outpatient antibiotic use in Europe and association with resistance: a cross-national database study.** *Lancet*. 365(9459):579–87.
35. **Vital signs: Overdoses of prescription opioid pain relievers and other drugs among women—United States, 1999–2010.** Centers for Disease Control and Prevention: Morbidity and Mortality Weekly Report (MMWR). 2013;62(26):537–42. http://www.cdc.gov/mmwr.
36. Ibid.
37. **Variation in Surgical Procedures.** Dartmouth Institute for Health Policy and Clinical Practice: Dartmouth Atlas of Health Care. 2014. http://www.dartmouthatlas.org/pages/variation_surgery_2.
38. Ibid.
39. Rosenthal, E. **After Surgery, Surprise $117,000 Medical Bill From Doctor He Didn't Know.** *New York Times*. September 20, 2014. http://www.nytimes.com/2014/09/21/us/drive-by-doctoring-surprise-medical-bills.html?hp&action=click&pgtype=Homepage&version=LedeSum&module=first-column-region®ion=top-news&WT.nav=top-news&_r=0.
40. Keeney BJ, et al. **Early predictors of lumbar spine surgery after occupational back injury: results from a prospective study of workers in Washington State.** *Spine* (Phila., Pa., 1976). May 15, 2013;38(11):953–64.
41. Willems P. **Decision making in surgical treatment of chronic low back pain: the performance of prognostic tests to select patients for lumbar spinal fusion.** *Acta Orthop Suppl*. February 2013;84(349):1–35.
42. Goldman L, Ausiello D. ***Cecil's Textbook of Medicine.*** New York, NY: Elsevier Press; 2004.
43. Institute of Medicine. ***Learning What Works Best: The Nation's Need for Evidence on Comparative Effectiveness in Health Care.*** 2007. http://www.ncbi.nlm.nih.gov/books/NBK64784/; reference list, http://www.ncbi.nlm.nih.gov/books/NBK50885/.
44. Kumar S, Nash DB. ***Demand Better! Revive Our Broken Healthcare System.*** Bozeman, MT: Second River Healthcare Press; 2011.
45. Hanney SR, et al. **How long does biomedical research take? Studying the time taken between biomedical and health research and its translation into products, policy, and practice.** *Health Res Policy Syst*. January 1, 2015;13:1.
46. Westfall J, Mold J, Fagnan L. **Practice-based research—"Blue Highways" on the NIH roadmap.** *JAMA*. 2007;297:403–6.
47. Trochim W. **Translation Won't Happen Without Dissemination and Implementation: Some Measurement and Evaluation Issues.** 3rd Annual Conference on the Science of Dissemination and Implementation. Bethesda, MD. 2010.
48. Green L, et al. **Diffusion theory and knowledge dissemination, utilization, and integration in public health.** *Annu Rev Public Health*. 2009;30:151–74.
49. Balas EA. **From appropriate care to evidence-based medicine.** *Pediatr Ann*. September 1998;27(9):581–84.
50. Ioannidis JA. **Contradicted and initially stronger effects in highly cited clinical research.** *JAMA*. 2005;294(2):218–28.

51. Pusztai L, Hatzis C, Andre F. **Reproducibility of research and preclinical validation: Problems and solutions.** *Nat Rev Clin Oncol.* December 2013;10(12):720–24.
52. Prinz F, Schlange T, Asadullah K. **Believe it or not: How much can we rely on published data on potential drug targets?** *Nat Rev Drug Discov.* August 2011;10(9):712.
53. Collins FS, Tabak LA. **Policy: NIH plans to enhance reproducibility.** Nature. January 30, 2014;505(7485):612-13.
54. Open Science Collaboration. **Estimating the reproducibility of psychological science.** *Science.* August 28, 2015: 349(6251), aac4716.
55. Prior JA, Silberstein JS, Stang J, eds. ***Physical Diagnosis: The History and Examination of the Patient***, 6th ed. St. Louis, MO: Mosby-Year Book; 1981: 7.
56. DeGowin EL, DeGowin RL. ***Bedside Diagnostic Examination.*** New York, NY: Macmillan; 1965.
57. Simel DL, Rennie D, Keitz SA, eds. ***The Rational Clinical Examination.*** New York, NY: McGraw-Hill; 2009: xiii.
58. DeGowin EL, DeGowin RL. ***Bedside Diagnostic Examination.*** New York, NY: Macmillan; 1965.
59. Simel DL, Rennie D, Keitz SA, eds. ***The Rational Clinical Examination.*** New York, NY: McGraw-Hill; 2009: xiii.
60. Paauw DS, et al. **Ability of primary care physicians to recognize physical findings associated with HIV infection.** *JAMA.* 1995;274:1380–82.
61. Mangione S, Nieman LZ. **Cardiac auscultatory skills of internal medicine and family practice trainees.** *JAMA.* 1997;278(9):717–22.
62. Ozuah PO, Dinkevich E. **Physical examination skills of US and international medical graduates.** *JAMA.* 2001;286(9):1021.
63. Anderson RC, Fagan MJ, Sebastian J. **Teaching students the art and science of physical diagnosis.** *Am J Med.* 2001;110(5):419–23.
64. Kohn LT, Corrigan JM, Donaldson MS, Committee on Quality of Health Care in America, Institute of Medicine, eds. ***To Err Is Human: Building a Safer Health System.*** Washington, DC: National Academies Press; 2000.
65. Smith M, et al. ***Best Care at Lower Cost: The Path to Continuously Learning Health Care in America.*** Washington, DC: National Academies Press; 2012.
66. Campbell EG, et al. **Professionalism in medicine: Results of a national survey of physicians.** *Ann Intern Med.* December 2007;147(11):795–803.
67. Lehnert BE, Bree RL. **Analysis of appropriateness of outpatient CT and MRI referred from primary care clinics at an academic medical center: how critical is the need for improved decision support.** *J Am Coll Radiol* 2010;7:192–97.
68. Rosenthal DI, et al. **Radiology order entry with decision support: initial clinical experiences.** *J Am Coll Radiol* 2006;3:799–806.
69. Bunt CW, et al. **Point-of-Care Estimated Radiation Exposure and Imaging Guidelines Can Reduce Pediatric Radiation Burden.** *J Am Board Fam Med.* May–June 2015;28:343–50.
70. U.S. Food and Drug Administration. **What Are the Radiation Risks from CT?** http://www.fda.gov/Radiation-EmittingProducts/RadiationEmittingProductsandProcedures/MedicalImaging/MedicalX-Rays/ucm115329.htm.
71. Cosgrove, James C. ***Physician Self-Referral: Recent Research from the Government Accountability Office (GAO).*** National Health Policy Forum. July 18, 2014.
72. Ibid.
73. Kirkner RM. **The Enduring Temptation of Physician Self-Referral.** *Managed Care.* October 2011. http://www.managedcaremag.com/content/enduring-temptation-physician-self-referral.
74. Ibid.
75. Cosgrove James C. ***Physician Self-Referral: Recent Research from the Government Accountability Office (GAO).*** National Health Policy Forum. July 18, 2014.
76. Kohn LT, Corrigan JM, Donaldson MS, Committee on Quality of Health Care in America, Institute of Medicine, eds. ***To Err Is Human: Building a Safer Health System.*** Washington, DC: National Academies Press; 2000.
77. Smith M, et al. ***Best Care at Lower Cost: The Path to Continuously Learning Health Care in America.*** Washington, DC: National Academies Press; 2012.
78. Campbell EG, et al. **Professionalism in medicine: Results of a national survey of physicians.** *Ann Intern Med.* December 2007;147(11):795–803.
79. Hartzband P, Groopman J. **How Medical Care Is Being Corrupted.** *New York Times.* November 18, 2014. http://www.nytimes.com/2014/11/19/opinion/how-medical-care-is-being-

corrupted.html?hp&action=click&pgtype=Homepage&module=c-column-top-span-region®ion=c-column-top-span-region&WT.nav=c-column-top-span-region&_r=1.
80. Ibid.
81. Taffel SM, Placek PJ, Liss T. **Trends in the United States cesarean section rate and reasons for the 1980–85 rise.** *Am J Public Health.* 1987;77:955–59.
82. Martin JA, et al. **Births: Final data for 2009.** *Natl Vital Stat Rep.* 2011;60:1–70.
83. Declercq ER, et al. **Listening to Mothers II: Report of the Second National U.S. Survey of Women's Childbearing Experiences.** Conducted January–February 2006 for Childbirth Connection by Harris Interactive in partnership with Lamaze International. *J Perinat Educ.* 2007;16:9–14.
84. Taffel SM, Placek PJ, Liss T. **Trends in the United States cesarean section rate and reasons for the 1980–85 rise.** *Am J Public Health.* 1987;77:955–59.
85. Ibid.
86. Martin JA, et al. **Births: Final data for 2009.** *Natl Vital Stat Rep.* 2011;60:1–70.
87. Declercq ER, et al. **Listening to Mothers II: Report of the Second National U.S. Survey of Women's Childbearing Experiences.** Conducted January–February 2006 for Childbirth Connection by Harris Interactive in partnership with Lamaze International. *J Perinat Educ.* 2007;16:9–14.
88. Ibid.
89. Bergstrom A, et al. **Establishment of intestinal microbiota during early life: A longitudinal, explorative study of a large cohort of Danish infants.** *Applied and Environmental Microbiology.* 2014;80(9):2889.
90. Ibid.
91. Moon C, et al. **Vertically transmitted faecal IgA levels determine extra-chromosomal phenotypic variation.** *Nature.* 2015.
92. Bergstrom A, et al. **Establishment of intestinal microbiota during early life: A longitudinal, explorative study of a large cohort of Danish infants.** *Applied and Environmental Microbiology.* 2014;80(9):2889.
93. Khafipour E, Ghia JE. **Mode of delivery and inflammatory disorders.** *J Immunol Clin Res.* 2013;1:1004.
94. Hansen CH, et al. **Mode of delivery shapes gut colonization pattern and modulates regulatory immunity in mice.** *J Immunol.* August 1, 2014;193(3):1213–22.
95. Vehik K, Dabelea, D. **Why are C-section deliveries linked to childhood type 1 diabetes?** *Diabetes.* 2012;61(1):36–37.
96. Adler SA, Wong-Kee-You, AMB. **Differential attentional responding in caesarean versus vaginally delivered infants.** *Attention, Perception, & Psychophysics.* August 11, 2015.
97. Kohn LT, Corrigan JM, Donaldson MS, Committee on Quality of Health Care in America, Institute of Medicine, eds. ***To Err Is Human: Building a Safer Health System.*** Washington, DC: National Academies Press; 2000.
98. Smith M, et al. ***Best Care at Lower Cost: The Path to Continuously Learning Health Care in America.*** Washington, DC: National Academies Press; 2012.
99. Campbell EG, et al. **Professionalism in medicine: Results of a national survey of physicians.** *Ann Intern Med.* December 2007;147(11):795–803.
100. Squires D. **Explaining high health care spending in the United States: An international comparison of supply, utilization, prices, and quality.** Commonwealth Fund. May 2012. http://www.commonwealthfund.org/~/media/Files/Publications/Issue percent20Brief/2012/May/1595_Squires_explaining_high_hlt_care_spending_intl_brief.pdf.
101. **Where Do You Get the Most for Your Health Care Dollar?** Bloomberg: Bloomberg Visual Data. September 18, 2014. http://www.bloomberg.com/infographics/2014-09-15/most-efficient-health-care-around-the-world.html.
102. Yong PL, Saunders RS, Olsen L, eds. ***The Healthcare Imperative: Lowering Costs and Improving Outcomes.*** Workshop series summary. Institute of Medicine of the National Academies. Washington, DC: National Academies Press; 2010.
103. U.S. Food and Drug Administration. **Medication Guides.** http://www.fda.gov/Drugs/DrugSafety/ucm085729.htm.

Chapter 3: Can't Stomach It?

1. Laugier R, et al. **Changes in pancreatic exocrine secretion with age: Pancreatic exocrine secretion does decrease in the elderly.** *Digestion.* 1991;50(3–4):202–11.
2. Morley JE. **The aging gut: Physiology.** *Clin Geriatr Med.* November 2007;23(4):757–67.
3. Grossman MI, Kirsner JB, Gillespie IE. **Basal and histalog-stimulated gastric secretion in control subjects and in**

patients with peptic ulcer or gastric cancer. *Gastroenterology*. 1963;45:15–26.

4. Krasinski SD, et al. **Fundic atrophic gastritis in an elderly population. Effect on hemoglobin and several serum nutritional indicators.** *J Am Geriatr Soc.* November 1986;34(11):800–06.
5. Heidelbaugh JJ, et al. **Overutilization of proton pump inhibitors: What the clinician needs to know.** *Therap Adv Gastroenterol.* July 2012;5(4):219–32.
6. Fohl AL, Regal RE. **Proton pump inhibitor-associated pneumonia: Not a breath of fresh air after all?** *World J Gastrointest Pharmacol Ther*. June 2011;2(3):17–26.
7. Ibid.
8. **Proton pump inhibitors: Use in adults.** Centers for Medicare & Medicaid Services. http://www.cms.gov/Medicare-Medicaid-Coordination/Fraud-Prevention/Medicaid-Integrity-Education/Pharmacy-Education-Materials/Downloads/ppi-adult-factsheet.pdf. Updated June 10, 2014.
9. **Clostridium difficile-associated diarrhea can be associated with stomach acid drugs known as proton pump inhibitors (PPIs).** U.S. Food and Drug Administration: FDA Drug Safety Communication. http://www.fda.gov/drugs/drugsafety/ucm290510.htm. Updated February 15, 2013.
10. Pali-Schöll I, et al. **Antacids and dietary supplements with an influence on the gastric pH increase the risk for food sensitization.** *Clin Exp Allergy*. July 2010;40(7):1091–98.
11. McColl K. **Effect of proton pump inhibitors on vitamins and iron.** *Am J Gastroenterol.* March 2009;104:S5–S9.
12. Frewin R, Henson A, Provan D. **ABC of clinical haematology. Iron deficiency anaemia.** *BMJ*. February 1997;314(7077):360–63.
13. Raffin SB, et al. **Intestinal absorption of hemoglobin iron-heme cleavage by mucosal heme oxygenase.** *J Clin Invest*. December 1974;54(6):1344–52.
14. Smith AD, et al. **Homocysteine-lowering by B vitamins slows the rate of accelerated brain atrophy in mild cognitive impairment: a randomized controlled trial.** *PLoS One*. September 8, 2010;5(9):e12244.
15. Douaud G, et al. **Preventing Alzheimer's disease–related gray matter atrophy by B-vitamin treatment.** *Proc Natl Acad Sci USA.* June 4, 2013;110(23):9523–28.
16. Barreras RF, Donaldson RM, Jr. **Effects of induced hypercalcemia on human gastric secretion.** *Gastroenterology*. 1967;52:670–75.
17. Levant JA, Walsh JH, Isenberg JI. **Stimulation of gastric secretion and gastrin release by single oral doses of calcium carbonate in man.** *N Engl J Med*. 1973;289:555–58.
18. Reeder DD, Conlee JL, Thompson JC. **Calcium carbonate antacid and serum gastrin concentration in duodenal ulcer.** *Surg Forum*. 1971;22:308–10.
19. Bradley PR, ed. ***British Herbal Compendium (Vol. 1): A handbook of scientific information on widely used plant drugs.*** Guilford and King's Lynn, Great Britain: Biddles Ltd.; 1992: 109–11.
20. Tan BKH, Vanitha J. **Immunomodulatory and antimicrobial effects of some traditional Chinese medicinal herbs: a review.** *Current Medicinal Chemistry*. June 2004;11(11):1423–30.
21. Ho JW, Jie M. **Pharmacological activity of cardiovascular agents from herbal medicine.** *Cardiovascular & Hematological Agents in Medicinal Chemistry* (formerly *Current Medicinal Chemistry—Cardiovascular & Hematological Agents*). October 2007;5(4):273–77.
22. Patwardhan B. **Ethnopharmacology and drug discovery.** *J Ethnopharmacol*. August 22, 2005;100(1–2):50–52.
23. Raja MKMM, Sethiya NK, Mishra SH. **A comprehensive review on *Nymphaea stellata*: A traditionally used bitter.** *J Adv Pharm Tech Res*. 2010;1(3):311–19.
24. Suryawanshi JAS. **An overview of *Citrus aurantium* used in treatment of various diseases.** *African Journal of Plant Science*. July 2011;5(7):390–95.
25. Aggarwal BB, Shishodia S. **Suppression of the nuclear factor-kappaB activation pathway by spice-derived phytochemicals: Reasoning for seasoning.** *Ann NY Acad Sci*. December 2004;1030:434–41. Review.
26. Kim MH, Kim SH, Yang WM. **Mechanisms of Action of Phytochemicals from Medicinal Herbs in the Treatment of Alzheimer's Disease.** *Planta Med*. October 2014;80(15):1249–58.
27. Jadeja R, Devkar RV, Nammi S. **Herbal medicines for the treatment of nonalcoholic steatohepatitis: current scenario and future prospects.** *Evid Based Complement Alternat Med*. 2014;2014:648308.
28. Wagner AE, Terschluesen AM, Rimbach G. **Health promoting effects of brassica-derived phytochemicals: From chemopreventive and anti-inflammatory activities to epigenetic regulation.** *Oxid Med Cell Longev*. 2013;2013:964539.

29. Gupta S, et al. **Garlic: An Effective Functional Food to Combat the Growing Antimicrobial Resistance.** *Pertanika Journal of Tropical Agricultural Science.* 2015;38(2):271–78.
30. Ibid.
31. Johns CE, et al. **The diurnal rhythm of the cytoprotective human trefoil protein TFF2 is reduced by factors associated with gastric mucosal damage: ageing, Helicobacter pylori infection, and sleep deprivation.** *Am J Gastroenterol.* July 2005;100(7):1491–97.
32. Semple J, et al. **Dramatic diurnal variation in the concentration of the human trefoil peptide TFF2 in gastric juice.** *Gut.* May 2001;48(5):648–55.

Chapter 4: Exploring Your Body's Connections

1. Bercik P, et al. **The intestinal microbiota affect central levels of brain-derived neurotropic factor and behavior in mice.** *Gastroenterology.* August 2011;141(2):599–609.
2. Rao AV, et al. **A randomized, double-blind, placebo-controlled pilot study of a probiotic in emotional symptoms of chronic fatigue syndrome.** *Gut Pathog.* March 2009;1(1):6.
3. Bercik P, et al. **The anxiolytic effect of Bifidobacterium longum NCC3001 involves vagal pathways for gut-brain communication.** *Neurogastroenterol Motil.* December 2011;23(12):1132–39.
4. Svensson E, et al. **Vagotomy and Subsequent Risk of Parkinson's Disease.** *Ann Neurol.* May 29, 2015. (Epub ahead of print.) PubMed PMID: 26031848.
5. Khalesi S, et al. **Effect of probiotics on blood pressure: A systematic review and meta-analysis of randomized, controlled trials.** *Hypertension.* Published online before print July 21, 2014.
6. DiRienzo DB. **Effect of probiotics on biomarkers of cardiovascular disease: Implications for heart-healthy diets.** *Nutrition Reviews.* January 2014;72(1):18–29.
7. Fabian E, Elmadfa I. **Influence of daily consumption of probiotic and conventional yoghurt on the plasma lipid profile in young healthy women.** *Ann Nutr Metab.* 2006;50:387–93.
8. Bongers G, et al. **Interplay of host microbiota, genetic perturbations, and inflammation promotes local development of intestinal neoplasms in mice.** *J Exp Med.* March 3, 2014;211(3):457–72.
9. Forli, L, et al. **Dietary vitamin K2 supplement improves bone status after lung and heart transplantation.** *Transplantation.* February 27, 2010;89(4):458–64.
10. Vermeer C, et al. **Beyond deficiency: Potential benefits of increased intakes of vitamin K for bone and vascular health.** *Eur J Nutr.* December 2004;43(6):325–35. Epub February 5, 2004. PubMed PMID: 15309455. Review.
11. Iwamoto J, et al. **Bone quality and vitamin K2 in type 2 diabetes: Review of preclinical and clinical studies.** *Nutr Rev.* March 2011;69(3):162–67.
12. Choi, HJ, et al. **Vitamin K2 Supplementation Improves Insulin Sensitivity via Osteocalcin Metabolism: A Placebo-Controlled Trial.** *Diabetes Care.* 2011;34(9):e147.
13. Varsha MK, et al. **Vitamin K1 alleviates streptozotocin-induced type 1 diabetes by mitigating free radical stress, as well as inhibiting NF-κB activation and iNOS expression in rat pancreas.** *Nutrition.* January 2015;31(1):214–22.
14. Veldhuis-Vlug AG, Fliers E, Bisschop PH. **Bone as a regulator of glucose metabolism.** *Neth J Med.* October 2013;71(8):396–400. Review.
15. Hart R, Doherty D. **The Potential Implications of a PCOS Diagnosis on a Woman's Long-Term Health Using Data Linkage.** *Journal of Clinical Endocrinology & Metabolism.* 2015;100(3):911–19.
16. Dunaif A, Fauser BC. **Renaming PCOS—a two-state solution.** *J Clin Endocrinol Metab.* 2013;98(11):4325.
17. Chang L. **Brain responses to visceral and somatic stimuli in irritable bowel syndrome: A central nervous system disorder?** *Gastroenterol Clin North Am.* June 2005;34(2):271–79.
18. Hang CH, et al. **Alterations of intestinal mucosa structure and barrier function following traumatic brain injury in rats.** *World J Gastroenterol.* December 9, 2003(12):2776–81.
19. Geissler A, et al. **Focal white-matter lesions in brain of patients with inflammatory bowel disease.** *Lancet.* April 8, 1995;345(8954):897–98.
20. Roman-Garcia P, et al. **Vitamin B12–dependent taurine synthesis regulates growth and bone mass.** *J Clin Invest.* July 1, 2014;124(7):2988–3002.
21. Iwamoto J, et al. **Bone quality and vitamin K2 in type 2 diabetes: Review of preclinical and clinical studies.** *Nutr Rev.* March 2011;69(3):162–67.

22. Sebastian A, et al. **The evolution-informed optimal dietary potassium intake of human beings greatly exceeds current and recommended intakes.** *Semin Nephrol.* November 2006;26:447–53.

23. König D, et al. **Effect of a Supplement Rich in Alkaline Minerals on Acid-Base Balance in Humans.** *Nutrition Journal.* June 10, 2009;8:23.

24. Sebastian A, et al. **The evolution-informed optimal dietary potassium intake of human beings greatly exceeds current and recommended intakes.** *Semin Nephrol.* November 2006;26:447–53.

25. Green DM, et al. **Serum potassium level and dietary potassium intake as risk factors for stroke.** *Neurology.* August 13, 2002;59(3):314–20.

26. Khaw KT, Barrett-Connor E. **Dietary potassium and stroke-associated mortality. A 12-year prospective population study.** *N Engl J Med.* January 29, 1987;316(5):235–40.

27. Green DM, et al. **Serum potassium level and dietary potassium intake as risk factors for stroke.** *Neurology.* August 13, 2002;59(3):314–20.

28. Khaw KT, Barrett-Connor E. **Dietary potassium and stroke-associated mortality. A 12-year prospective population study.** *N Engl J Med.* January 29, 1987;316(5):235–40.

29. Park YG, Moon JH, Park SY. **Lactoferrin from bovine colostrum regulates prolyl hydroxylase 2 activity and prevents prion protein-mediated neuronal cell damage via cellular prion protein.** *Neuroscience.* August 22, 2014;274:187–97.

30. Rai D, et al. **Longitudinal changes in lactoferrin concentrations in human milk: a global systematic review.** *Crit Rev Food Sci Nutr.* 2014;54(12):1539–47.

31. Wang J, et al. **Recombination adenovirus-mediated human lactoferrin cDNA inhibits the growth of human MCF-7 breast cancer cells.** *J Pharm Pharmacol.* March 2012;64(3):457–63.

32. Kanwar JR, et al. **Fe-bLf nanoformulation targets surviving to kill colon cancer stem cells and maintains absorption of iron, calcium and zinc.** *Nanomedicine* (Lond). January 2015;10(1):35–55.

33. Gibbons JA, Kanwar RK, Kanwar JR. **Lactoferrin and cancer in different cancer models.** *Front Biosci* (Schol Ed). June 1, 2011;3:1080–8. Review.

34. Lönnerdal B. **Nutritional roles of lactoferrin.** *Curr Opin Clin Nutr Metab Care.* May 2009;12(3):293–97.

35. Tian H, et al. **Evaluation of the cytoprotective effects of bovine lactoferrin against intestinal toxins using cellular model systems.** *Biometals.* June 2010;23(3):589–92.

36. Guttner, Y, et al. **Human recombinant lactoferrin is ineffective in the treatment of human Helicobacter pylori infection.** *Alimentary Pharmacology & Therapeutics.* 2003;125–29.

37. Amini AA, Nair LS. **Lactoferrin: a biologically active molecule for bone regeneration.** *Curr Med Chem.* 2011;18(8):1220–9. Review.

38. Naot D, et al. **Lactoferrin—a novel bone growth factor.** *Clin Med Res.* May 2005;3(2):93–101. Review.

39. Cornish J, et al. **Lactoferrin and bone; structure-activity relationships.** *Biochem Cell Biol.* June 2006;84(3):297–302.

40. Włodarski KH, et al. **[The importance of lactoferrin in bone regeneration]**. *Pol Merkur Lekarski.* July 2014;37(217):65–67. Review. Polish.

41. Cornish J, et al. **Lactoferrin is a potent regulator of bone cell activity and increases bone formation in vivo.** *Endocrinology.* September 2004;145(9):4366–74.

42. Andrews PW, et al. **Is serotonin an upper or a downer? The evolution of the serotonergic system and its role in depression and the antidepressant response**. *Neuroscience & Biobehavioral Reviews.* 2015; 51:164.

43. Nagahara N, et al. **Antioxidant enzyme, 3-mercaptopyruvate sulfurtransferase—knockout mice exhibit increased anxiety-like behaviors: A model for human mercaptolactate-cysteine disulfiduria.** *Sci Rep.* 2013;3:1986.

44. Branchi I. **The double edged sword of neural plasticity: increasing serotonin levels leads to both greater vulnerability to depression and improved capacity to recover.** *Psychoneuroendocrinology.* April 2011;36(3):339–51.

45. Morley WA, Seneff S. **Diminished brain resilience syndrome: A modern day neurological pathology of increased susceptibility to mild brain trauma, concussion, and downstream neurodegeneration.** *Surg Neurol Int.* 2014;5:97.

46. Connor KM, Davidson JR, Churchill LE. **Adverse-effect profile of kava.** *CNS Spectr.* October 2001;6(10):848, 850–53.

47. Alpert JE, Fava M. **Nutrition and depression: the role of folate.** *Nutrition Reviews.* May 1997;55(5):145–49.

48. Feighner JP, Brown SL, Olivier JE. **Electrosleep therapy: a controlled double blind study.** *Journal of Nervous and Mental Disease.* 1973;157(2):121–28.

49. Pozos RS, et al. **Electrosleep versus electroconvulsive therapy.** In Reynolds DV, Sjorberg AE, eds. *Neuroelectric Research.* Springfield, IL: Charles Thomas; 1971: 221–25.

50. Rosenthal SH, Wulfsohn NL. **Studies of electrosleep with active and simulated treatment.** *Current Therapeutic Research*. 1970;12(3):126–30.
51. Schmitt R, Capo T, Boyd E. **Cranial electrotherapy stimulation as a treatment for anxiety in chemically dependent persons.** *Alcoholism: Clinical and Experimental Research*. 1986;10(2):158–60.
52. Shealy CN, et al. **Depression: a diagnostic, neurochemical profile and therapy with cranial electrical stimulation (CES).** *Journal of Neurological and Orthopaedic Medicine and Surgery*. 1989;10(4):319–21.
53. Weiss MF. **The treatment of insomnia through the use of electrosleep: an EEG study.** *Journal of Nervous and Mental Disease*. 1973;157(2):108–20.
54. Berg K, Siever D. **Audio-Visual Entrainment (AVE) as a treatment modality for seasonal affective disorder.** *Journal of Neurotherapy*. 2009;13(3):166–75.
55. Joyce M, Siever D. **Audio-Visual Entrainment (AVE) Program as a Treatment for Behavior Disorders in a School Setting.** From the appendices of ***The Rediscovery of Audio-Visual Entrainment Technology***, by D. Siever. C.E.T. 1997. https://mindalive.com/index.cfm/research/add-adhd/audio-visual-entrainment-ave-program-as-a-treatment-for-behavior-disorders-in-a-school-setting-michael-joyce-dave-siever/.
56. Budzynski T, Budzynski H, Tang J. **Biolight effects on the EEG.** *SynchroMed Report*. 1998. Seattle, WA.
57. Berg K, Siever D. **Outcome of medical methods, audio-visual entrainment, and nutritional supplementation for fibromyalgia syndrome: A pilot study.** 1999. Unpublished manuscript.
58. Berg K, et al. **Outcome of Medical Methods, Audio-Visual Entrainment (AVE) and Nutritional Supplementation for the Treatment of Fibromyalgia Syndrome.** http://www.mindmods.com/resources/Study-Fibromyalgia.html. From the appendices of ***The Rediscovery of Audio-Visual Entrainment Technology***, by D. Siever. C.E.T. 1997. https://mindalive.com/index.cfm/research/add-adhd/audio-visual-entrainment-ave-program-as-a-treatment-for-behavior-disorders-in-a-school-setting-michael-joyce-dave-siever/.
59. Trudeau D. **A trial of 18 Hz audio-visual stimulation on attention and concentration in chronic fatigue syndrome (CFS).** *Proceedings of the Annual Conference for the International Society for Neuronal Regulation*. 1999.
60. Joyce M, Siever D. **Audio-visual entrainment program as a treatment for behavior disorders in a school setting.** *Journal of Neurotherapy*. 2000;4(2):9–15.
61. Wolitzky-Taylor KB, Telch MJ. **Efficacy of self-administered treatments for pathological academic worry: A randomized controlled trial.** *Behaviour Research and Therapy*. 2010;48:840–50.
62. Shelby G, et al. **Functional Abdominal Pain in Childhood and Long-term Vulnerability to Anxiety Disorders.** *Pediatrics*. September 1, 2013;132(3):475–82. http://pediatrics.aappublications.org/content/132/3/475.full.
63. Cryan JF, O'Mahony SM. **The microbiome-gut-brain axis: from bowel to behavior.** *Neurogastroenterol Motil*. March 2011;23(3):187–92.
64. Foster JA, McVey K-A. **Gut–brain axis: how the microbiome influences anxiety and depression.** *Trends in Neurosciences*. May 2013;36(5):305–12.
65. Chassaing B, et al. **Dietary emulsifiers impact the mouse gut microbiota promoting colitis and metabolic syndrome.** *Nature*, 2015.
66. De Lorgeril M, Salen P. **Gluten and wheat intolerance today: Are modern wheat strains involved?** *Int J Food Sci Nutr*. August 2014;65(5):577–81.
67. Pizzuti D, et al. **Lack of intestinal mucosal toxicity of *Triticum monococcum* in celiac disease patients.** *Scand J Gastroenterol*. November 2006;41(11):1305–11.
68. Ibid.
69. Vincentini O, et al. **Environmental factors of celiac disease: cytotoxicity of hulled wheat species Triticum monococcum, T. turgidum ssp. dicoccum and T. aestivum ssp. spelta.** *J Gastroenterol Hepatol*. November 2007;22(11):1816–22.
70. Kasarda DD. **Triticum moncoccum and celiac disease.** *Scand J Gastroenterol*. September 2007;42(9):1141–42; author reply 1143–44.
71. Spaenij-Dekking L, et al. **Natural variation in toxicity of wheat: Potential for selection of nontoxic varieties for celiac disease patients.** *Gastroenterology*. September 2005;129(3):797–806.
72. De Vincenzi M, et al. **In vitro toxicity testing of alcohol-soluble proteins from diploid wheat Triticum monococcum in celiac disease.** *Biochem Toxicol*. 1996;11:313–18.
73. Hadjivassiliou M, Grunewald RA, Davies-Jones GA. **Gluten sensitivity as a neurological illness.** *J Neurosurg Psychiatry*,

2002 May; 72(5):560-563.

74. Perry GH, et al. **Diet and the evolution of human amylase gene copy number variation.** *Nature genetics*. 2007;39(10):1256–60.
75. Lee C, et al. **CNVs vs. SNPs: Understanding Human Structural Variation in Disease.** Webinar. Science/AAAS. July 16, 2008. http://webinar.sciencemag.org/webinar/archive/cnvs-vs-snps.
76. Ibid.
77. Samsel A, Seneff S. **Glyphosate, pathways to modern diseases II: Celiac sprue and gluten intolerance.** *Interdiscip Toxicol.* December 2013;6(4):159–84.
78. Carman JA, et al. **A long-term toxicology study on pigs fed a combined genetically modified (GM) soy and GM maize diet.** *J Organ Syst.* 2013;8:38–54.51.
79. Shehata AA, et al. **The effect of glyphosate on potential pathogens and beneficial members of poultry microbiota *in vitro*.** *Curr Microbiol.* 2013;66:350–58.
80. Fernandez-Cornejo J, et al. **Pesticide Use in U.S. Agriculture: 21 Selected Crops, 1960–2008.** U.S. Department of Agriculture, Economic Research Service. Economic Information Bulletin No. 124. May 2014.
81. U.S. Environmental Protection Agency. **2007 Pesticide Market Estimates.**
82. Rao AV, et al. **A randomized, double-blind, placebo-controlled pilot study of a probiotic in emotional symptoms of chronic fatigue syndrome.** *Gut Pathog*. March 2009;1(1):6.
83. Bercik P, et al. **The anxiolytic effect of Bifidobacterium longum NCC3001 involves vagal pathways for gut-brain communication.** *Neurogastroenterol Motil*. December 2011;23(12):1132–39.

Chapter 5: Our Health in Pieces

1. Fox, K. **The Smell Report.** Social Issues Research Centre (SIRC). November 20, 2009. http://www.sirc.org/publik/smell_hist.html.
2. Inglis-Arkell E. **These diseases can be diagnosed by smell.** io9. November 12, 2012. http://io9.com/5959395/these-diseases-can-be-diagnosed-by-smell.
3. Bijland LR, Bomers MK, Smulders YM. **Smelling the diagnosis: a review on the use of scent in diagnosing disease.** *Neth J Med*. July–August 2013;71(6):300–307.
4. Balseiro SC, Correia HR. **Is olfactory detection of human cancer by dogs based on major histocompatibility complex-dependent odour components? A possible cure and a precocious diagnosis of cancer.** *Med Hypotheses*. 2006;66(2):270–72.
5. Horvath G, Andersson H, Nemes S. **Cancer odor in the blood of ovarian cancer patients: a retrospective study of detection by dogs during treatment, 3 and 6 months afterward.** *BMC Cancer*. August 2013;13:396.
6. American College of Cardiology. **Cardiologists Fail to Identify Basic and Advanced Murmurs.** http://www.acc.org/about-acc/press-releases/2015/08/31/10/14/cardiologists-fail-to-identify-basic-and-advanced-murmurs?w_nav=S.
7. Farrell PM, et al. **Guidelines for diagnosis of cystic fibrosis in newborns through older adults: cystic fibrosis consensus report.** *J Pediatr*. August 2008;153(2):S4–S14.
8. Quinton PM. **Cystic fibrosis: lessons from the sweat gland.** *Physiology*. June 2007;22:212–25.

Chapter 6: What Color Is Your Traffic Light?

1. Goode E. **Farmers Put Down the Plow for More Productive Soil.** *New York Times*. March 9, 2015. http://www.nytimes.com/2015/03/10/science/farmers-put-down-the-plow-for-more-productive soil.html.
2. **International Classification of Diseases (ICD).** World Health Organization. http://www.who.int/classifications/icd/en/. Updated 2010.
3. **Clinical Laboratory Statistics.** UCSD Lab Medicine. http://ucsdlabmed.wikidot.com/chapter-1. Updated April 19, 2010.
4. Markelonis G, Tae Hwan OH. **A sciatic nerve protein has a trophic effect on development and maintenance of skeletal muscle cells in culture.** *Proc Natl Acad Scie USA*. May 1979;76(5):2470–74.
5. Schwartz SM, Campbell GR, Campbell JH. **Replication of smooth muscle cells in vascular disease.** *Circ Res*. April 1986;58(4):427–44.
6. Kardami E, Spector D, Strohman RC. **Selected muscle and nerve extracts contain an activity which stimulates myoblast proliferation and which is distinct from transferrin.** *Dev Biol*. December 1985;112(2):353–58.

7. Helgren ME, et al. **Trophic effect of ciliary neurotrophic factor on denervated skeletal muscle.** *Cell.* February 1994;76(3):493–504.
8. Oh TH. **Neurotrophic effects of sciatic nerve extracts on muscle development in culture.** *Experimental Neurology.* February 1976;50(2):376–86.
9. Dale JM, et al. **The spinal muscular atrophy mouse model, SMAΔ7, displays altered axonal transport without global neurofilament alterations.** *Acta Neuropathology.* September 2011;122:331–41.
10. Inestrosa NC, Fernandez HL. **Muscle enzymatic changes induced by blockage of axoplasmic transport.** *J Neurophysiol.* November 1976;39(6):1236–45.
11. Moore AZ, et al. **Difference in muscle quality over the adult life span and biological correlates in the Baltimore Longitudinal Study of Aging.** *J Am Geriatr Soc.* February 2014;62(2):230–36.
12. Ward RE, et al. **Peripheral nerve function and lower extremity muscle power in older men.** *Arch Phys Med Rehabil.* April 2014;95(4):726–33.
13. Yamada M, et al. **Age-dependent changes in skeletal muscle mass and visceral fat area in Japanese adults from 40 to 79 years-of-age.** *Geriatr Gerontol Int.* February 2014;14(Suppl 1):8–14.
14. Tanimoto Y, et al. **Aging changes in muscle mass of Japanese.** *Nihon Ronen Igakkai Zasshi.* 2010;47(1):52–57.
15. **Clinical Laboratory Statistics.** UCSD Lab Medicine. http://ucsdlabmed.wikidot.com/chapter-1. Updated April 19, 2010.
16. Brook RD, et al. **Usefulness of visceral obesity (waist/hip ratio) in predicting vascular endothelial function in healthy overweight adults.** *American Journal of Cardiology.* 88(11):1264–69.

Chapter 7: The Power That Heals You

1. Breig A. ***Biomechanics of the central nervous system: Some basic normal and pathologic phenomena.*** Stockholm: Almqvist and Wiksell; 1960.
2. Shacklock M. ***Clinical Neurodynamics Course Manual.*** Neurodynamic Solutions NDS. Adelaide, Australia; 2007.
3. **SOTO USA** (Sacro Occipital Technique Organization). http://www.sotousa.com/wp.
4. **What Is Network Spinal Analysis?** Wise World Seminars. http://wiseworldseminars.com/network-spinal-analysis.
5. Yogananda P. ***Scientific Healing Affirmations.*** Los Angeles, CA: Self-Realization Fellowship; 1957: 31–32.2.
6. Mann F. ***Acupuncture: The Ancient Chinese Healing Art and How It Works Scientifically.*** New York, NY: Vintage Books; 1973.
7. Fauci AS, et al. ***Harrison's Principles of Internal Medicine***, 17th ed. New York, NY: McGraw-Hill Medical; 2008.
8. Bourane S, et al. **Identification of a spinal circuit for light touch and fine motor control.** *Cell.* 2015;160(3):503.
9. **Spinal cord processes information just as areas of brains do, research finds.** Queen's University: *ScienceDaily.* March 23, 2011. http://www.sciencedaily.com/releases/2011/03/110322151308.htm.
10. Andersen P, Andersson SA. ***Physiological Basis of the Alpha Rhythm.*** New York, NY: Appleton-Century-Crofts; 1968.
11. Davson H. ***A Textbook of General Physiology***, 4th ed. Baltimore, MD: Lippincott Williams & Wilkins; 1970: 559.
12. Destexhe A, Babloyantz A, Sejnowski TJ. **Ionic mechanisms for intrinsic slow oscillations in thalamic relay neurons.** *Biophys J.* October 1993;65(4):1538–52.
13. Wallenstein GV. **A model of the electrophysiological properties of nucleus reticularis thalami neurons.** *Biophys J.* April 1994;66:978–88.
14. Becker RO. **The machine brain and properties of the mind.** *Subtle Energies & Energy Medicine.* 1990;113:79–97.
15. Becker RO. ***Cross Current: The Perils of Electropollution.*** New York, NY: Tarcher; 1990.
16. Oschman JL. **What is healing energy? Part 3: Silent pulses.** *Journal of Bodywork and Movement Therapies.* April 1997;1(3):179–89.
17. Oschman JL. ***Energy Medicine: The Scientific Basis.*** London, UK: Churchill Livingstone; 2000.
18. Da Silva FL. **Neural mechanisms underlying brain waves: from neural membranes to networks.** *Electroencephalography and Clinical Neurophysiology.* August 1991;79(2):81–93.
19. Steriade M, Deschenes M. **The thalamus as a neuronal oscillator.** *Brain Research Reviews.* November 1984;8(1):1–63.
20. Hahn G, et al. **Communication through resonance in spiking neuronal networks.** *PLoS Computational Biology.* 2014;10(8).
21. Tchumatchenko T, Clopath C. **Oscillations emerging from noise-driven steady state in networks with electrical synapses and subthreshold resonance.** *Nature Communications.* 2014;5:5512.
22. Ibid.

23. Ibid.
24. Koch RS. **A somatic component in heart disease.** *J Am Osteopath Assoc.* May 1961;60:735–40.
25. Tashiro M, et al. **Cerebral metabolic changes in men after chiropractic spinal manipulation for neck pain.** *Altern Ther Health Med.* November–December 2011;17(6):12–17.
26. Hülse M. **Cervicogenic hearing loss.** *HNO.* October 1994;42(10):604–13. German.
27. Miller JE, Newell D, Bolton JE. **Efficacy of chiropractic manual therapy on infant colic: a pragmatic single-blind, randomized controlled trial.** *Journal of manipulative and physiological therapeutics.* 2012;35(8):600–607.
28. Takeda Y, Arai S. **Relationship Between Vertebral Deformities and Allergic Diseases.** *Internet Journal of Orthopedic Surgery.* 2003;2(1).
29. Qu L, et al. **Irritable bowel syndrome treated by traditional Chinese spinal orthopedic manipulation.** *J Tradit Chin Med.* December 2012;32(4):565–70.
30. Jørgensen LS, Fossgreen J. **Back pain and spinal pathology in patients with functional upper abdominal pain.** *Scand J Gastroenterol.* December 1990;25(12):1235–41.
31. Henderson CN. **The basis for spinal manipulation: chiropractic perspective of indications and theory.** *J Electromyogr Kinesiol.* October 2012;22(5):632–42.
32. Kangilaski J. **Chiropractic can involve more than spinal manipulation.** *Forum Med.* November 1978;1(8):33–35.
33. Hawk C, et al. **Chiropractic care for nonmusculoskeletal conditions: a systematic review with implications for whole systems research.** *J Altern Complement Med.* June 2007;13(5):491–512.. Review.
34. Orlin JR, Didriksen A. **Results of chiropractic treatment of lumbopelvic fixation in 44 patients admitted to an orthopedic department.** *J Manipulative Physiol Ther.* February 2007;30(2):135–39.
35. Melin T, Söderström A. **No proven connection between chiropractic neck manipulation and stroke.** *Lakartidningen.* May 30–June 3, 2007;104(22):1713; discussion 1713–14.
36. Gouveia LO, Castanho P, Ferreira JJ. **Safety of chiropractic interventions: a systematic review.** *Spine* (Phila Pa 1976). May 15, 2009;34(11):E405–13.
37. Ndetan H, et al. **The Role of Chiropractic Care in the Treatment of Dizziness or Balance Disorders: Analysis of National Health Interview Survey Data.** *J Evid Based Complementary Altern Med.* September 11, 2015. pii: 2156587215604974.
38. Mandolesi S, et al. **Preliminary results after upper cervical chiropractic care in patients with chronic cerebro-spinal venous insufficiency and multiple sclerosis.** *Ann Ital Chir.* May–June, 2015;86(3):192–200.
39. Pettigrew J. **Utilizing chiropractic for optimal pregnancy and birth outcomes.** *Midwifery Today Int Midwife.* Summer 2014;(110):56–57.
40. Peterson CK, Mühlemann D, Humphreys BK. **Outcomes of pregnant patients with low back pain undergoing chiropractic treatment: a prospective cohort study with short term, medium term and 1 year follow-up.** *Chiropr Man Therap.* April 1, 2014;22(1):15.
41. Weigel PA, et al. **The comparative effect of episodes of chiropractic and medical treatment on the health of older adults.** *J Manipulative Physiol Ther.* March–April, 2014;37(3):143–54.
42. Alcantara J, Alcantara JD, Alcantara J. **Chiropractic treatment for asthma? You bet!** *J Asthma.* June 2010;47(5):597–58.
43. Pickar JG. **Neurophysiological effects of spinal manipulation.** *Spine J.* September–October 2002;2(5):357–71. Review.
44. DeMaria A, et al. **A weight loss program in a chiropractic practice: a retrospective analysis.** *Complement Ther Clin Pract.* May 2014;20(2):125–29.
45. Peterson CK, Bolton J, Humphreys BK. **Predictors of improvement in patients with acute and chronic low back pain undergoing chiropractic treatment.** *J Manipulative Physiol Ther.* September 2012;35(7):525–33.
46. Marchand AM. **Chiropractic care of children from birth to adolescence and classification of reported conditions: an Internet cross-sectional survey of 956 European chiropractors.** *J Manipulative Physiol Ther.* June 2012;35(5):372–80.
47. Hurwitz EL. **Epidemiology: spinal manipulation utilization.** *J Electromyogr Kinesiol.* October 2012;22(5):648–54.
48. **Spinal manipulation and exercise trump drugs for neck pain.** *Harvard Women's Health Watch.* April 2012;19(8):6–7.
49. Miller JE, et al. **Contribution of chiropractic therapy to resolving suboptimal breastfeeding: a case series of 114 infants.** *J Manipulative Physiol Ther.* October 2009;32(8):670–74.
50. Goertz CM, et al. **Adding chiropractic manipulative therapy to standard medical care for patients with acute low back pain: results of a pragmatic randomized comparative effectiveness study.** *Spine* (Phila Pa 1976). April 15, 2013;38(8):627–34.

51. Smith DL, Cramer GD. **Spinal Manipulation Is Not an Emerging Risk Factor for Stroke Nor Is It Major Head/Neck Trauma. Don't Just Read the Abstract!** *Open Neurol J.* 2011;5:46–47.
52. Daligadu J, et al. **Alterations in cortical and cerebellar motor processing in subclinical neck pain patients following spinal manipulation.** *J Manipulative Physiol Ther.* October 2013;36(8):527–37.
53. Noudeh YJ, Vatankhah N, Baradaran HR. **Reduction of current migraine headache pain following neck massage and spinal manipulation.** *Int J Ther Massage Bodywork.* 2012;5(1):5–13. Epub 2012 Mar 31.
54. Bryans R, et al. **Evidence-based guidelines for the chiropractic treatment of adults with headache.** *J Manipulative Physiol Ther.* June 2011;34(5):274–89.
55. Ogura T, et al. **Cerebral metabolic changes in men after chiropractic spinal manipulation for neck pain.** *Altern Ther Health Med.* November–December 2011;17(6):12–17.
56. Kovanur Sampath K, et al. **Measureable changes in the neuro-endocrinal mechanism following spinal manipulation.** *Med Hypotheses.* October 10, 2015.
57. Stochkendahl MJ, et al. **Chiropractic treatment vs. self-management in patients with acute chest pain: a randomized controlled trial of patients without acute coronary syndrome.** *J Manipulative Physiol Ther.* January 2012;35(1):7–17.
58. Marchand AM. **A Literature Review of Pediatric Spinal Manipulation and Chiropractic Manipulative Therapy: Evaluation of Consistent Use of Safety Terminology.** *J Manipulative Physiol Ther.* August 27, 2012.
59. Cecchi F, et al. **Predictors of functional outcome in patients with chronic low back pain undergoing back school, individual physiotherapy or spinal manipulation.** *Eur J Phys Rehabil Med.* September 2012;48(3):371–78. Epub May 8, 2012.
60. Haavik H, Murphy B. **The role of spinal manipulation in addressing disordered sensorimotor integration and altered motor control.** *J Electromyogr Kinesiol.* October 2012;22(5):768–76.
61. Lehman G. **Kinesiological research: The use of surface electromyography for assessing the effects of spinal manipulation.** *J Electromyogr Kinesiol.* Oct 2012;22(5):692–96.
62. Leininger BD, Evans R, Bronfort G. **Exploring patient satisfaction: a secondary analysis of a randomized clinical trial of spinal manipulation, home exercise, and medication for acute and subacute neck pain.** *J Manipulative Physiol Ther.* October 2014;37(8):593–601.
63. Senna MK, Machaly SA. **Does maintained spinal manipulation therapy for chronic nonspecific low back pain result in better long-term outcome?** *Spine* (Phila Pa 1976). August 15, 2011;36(18):1427–37.
64. Herzog W, et al. **Vertebral artery strains during high-speed, low amplitude cervical spinal manipulation.** *J Electromyogr Kinesiol.* October 2012;22(5):740–46.
65. Walker BF, et al. **A Cochrane review of combined chiropractic interventions for low-back pain.** *Spine* (Phila Pa 1976). February 1, 2011;36(3):230–42.
66. Posadzki P. **Is spinal manipulation effective for pain? An overview of systematic reviews.** *Pain Med.* June 2012;13(6):754–61. doi: 10.1111/j.1526-4637.2012.01397.x. Epub 2012 May 23.
67. Roy RA, Boucher JP, Comtois AS. **Heart rate variability modulation after manipulation in pain-free patients vs. patients in pain.** *J Manipulative Physiol Ther.* May 2009;32(4):277–86.
68. Bolton PS, Budgell B. **Visceral responses to spinal manipulation.** *J Electromyogr Kinesiol.* October 2012;22(5):777–84.
69. Vieira-Pellenz F, et al. **Short-term effect of spinal manipulation on pain perception, spinal mobility, and full height recovery in male subjects with degenerative disk disease: a randomized controlled trial.** *Arch Phys Med Rehabil.* September 2014;95(9):1613–19.
70. Castro-Sánchez AM, et al. **Short-term effectiveness of spinal manipulative therapy versus functional technique in patients with chronic non-specific low back pain: a pragmatic randomized controlled trial.** *Spine J.* September 8, 2015. pii: S1529-9430(15)01363-7.
71. Plaza-Manzano G, et al. **Changes in biochemical markers of pain perception and stress response after spinal manipulation.** *J Orthop Sports Phys Ther.* April 2014;44(4):231–39.
72. Southerst D, et al. **The effectiveness of manual therapy for the management of musculoskeletal disorders of the upper and lower extremities: a systematic review by the Ontario Protocol for Traffic Injury Management (OPTIMa) Collaboration.** *Chiropr Man Therap.* October 27, 2015;23:30.
73. Koppenhaver SL, et al. **Association between history and physical examination factors and change in lumbar multifidus muscle thickness after spinal manipulation in patients with low back pain.** *J Electromyogr Kinesiol.* October 2012;22(5):724–31. doi: 10.1016/j.jelekin.2012.03.004. Epub 2012 Apr 18.

74. Tuchin P. **A replication of the study "Adverse effects of spinal manipulation: a systematic review."** *Chiropr Man Therap.* September 21, 2012;20(1):30. doi: 10.1186/2045-709X-20-30.

75. Molina-Ortega F, et al. **Immediate effects of spinal manipulation on nitric oxide, substance P and pain perception.** *Man Ther.* October 2014;19(5):411–17.

76. Nougarou F, et al. **Physiological responses to spinal manipulation therapy: investigation of the relationship between electromyographic responses and peak force.** *J Manipulative Physiol Ther.* November–December 2013;36(9):557–63. doi: 10.1016/j.jmpt.2013.08.006.

77. O'Neill S, Ødegaard-Olsen Ø, Søvde B. **The effect of spinal manipulation on deep experimental muscle pain in healthy volunteers.** *Chiropr Man Therap.* September 7, 2015;23:25.

78. Whedon JM, et al. **Risk of stroke after chiropractic spinal manipulation in Medicare B beneficiaries aged 66 to 99 years with neck pain.** *J Manipulative Physiol Ther.* February 2015;38(2):93–101.

79. Achalandabaso A, et al. **Tissue damage markers after a spinal manipulation in healthy subjects: a preliminary report of a randomized controlled trial.** *Dis Markers.* 2014;2014:815379. doi: 10.1155/2014/815379. Epub 2014 Dec 25.

80. Yuan WA, et al. **Effect of spinal manipulation on brain functional activity in patients with lumbar disc herniation.** *Zhejiang Da Xue Xue Bao Yi Xue Ban.* March 2015;44(2):124–30, 137.

81. Aoyagi M, et al. **Response to Letter to the Editor Re: "Determining the level of evidence for the effectiveness of spinal manipulation in the upper limb: A systematic review meta-analysis."** *Man Ther.* May 8, 2015. pii: S1356-689X(15)00071-5.

82. Petersen T, Christensen R, Juhl C. **Predicting a clinically important outcome in patients with low back pain following McKenzie therapy or spinal manipulation: a stratified analysis in a randomized controlled trial.** *BMC Musculoskelet Disord.* April 1, 2015;16:74.

83. Reed WR, et al. **Neural responses to the mechanical characteristics of high velocity, low amplitude spinal manipulation: Effect of specific contact site.** *Man Ther.* March 27, 2015. pii: S1356-689X(15)00061-2.

84. Niazi IK, et al. **Changes in H-reflex and V-waves following spinal manipulation.** *Exp Brain Res.* April 2015;233(4):1165–73.

85. Schneider M, et al. **Comparison of spinal manipulation methods and usual medical care for acute and subacute low back pain: a randomized clinical trial.** *Spine* (Phila Pa 1976). February 15, 2015;40(4):209–17.

86. Bronfort G, et al. **Spinal manipulation and home exercise with advice for subacute and chronic back-related leg pain: a trial with adaptive allocation.** *Ann Intern Med.* September 16, 2014;161(6):381–91.

87. Rodine RJ, Vernon H. **Cervical radiculopathy: a systematic review on treatment by spinal manipulation and measurement with the Neck Disability Index.** *J Can Chiropr Assoc.* March 2012;56(1):18–28.

88. Maiers M, et al. **Adverse events among seniors receiving spinal manipulation and exercise in a randomized clinical trial.** *Man Ther.* April 2015;20(2):335–41.

89. Bronfort G, et al. **Spinal manipulation, medication, or home exercise with advice for acute and subacute neck pain: a randomized trial.** *Ann Intern Med.* January 3, 2012;156(1 Pt 1):1–10.

90. Coronado RA, et al. **Changes in pain sensitivity following spinal manipulation: a systematic review and meta-analysis.** *J Electromyogr Kinesiol.* October 2012;22(5):752–67.

91. McMorland G, et al. **Manipulation or microdiskectomy for sciatica? A prospective randomized clinical study.** *J Manipulative Physiol Ther.* October 2010;33(8):576–84.

92. Wiberg JM, Nordsteen J, Nilsson N. **The short-term effect of spinal manipulation in the treatment of infantile colic: a randomized controlled clinical trial with a blinded observer.** *J Manipulative Physiol Ther.* October 1999;22(8):517–22.

93. Alcantara J, Alcantara JD, Alcantara J. **The chiropractic care of infants with colic: a systematic review of the literature.** *Explore* (NY). May–June 2011;7(3):168–74.

94. Lucassen P. **Colic in infants.** *BMJ Clin Evid.* February 5, 2010;2010. pii: 0309.

95. Strunk RG, Hawk C. **Effects of chiropractic care on dizziness, neck pain, and balance: a single-group, preexperimental, feasibility study.** *J Chiropr Med.* December 2009;8(4):156–64.

96. Hawk C, et al. **Best practices recommendations for chiropractic care for infants, children, and adolescents: results of a consensus process.** *J Manipulative Physiol Ther.* October 2009;32(8):639–47.

97. Hawk C, Cambron J. **Chiropractic care for older adults: effects on balance, dizziness, and chronic pain.** *J Manipulative Physiol Ther.* July–August 2009;32(6):431–37.

98. Stuber K, Sajko S, Kristmanson K. **Chiropractic treatment of lumbar spinal stenosis: a review of the literature.** *J Chiropr Med.* June 2009;8(2):77–85.

99. Williams NH, et al. **Psychological response in spinal manipulation (PRISM): a systematic review of psychological outcomes in randomised controlled trials.** *Complement Ther Med.* December 2007;15(4):271–83.

100. Boline PD, et al. **Spinal manipulation vs. amitriptyline for the treatment of chronic tension-type headaches: a randomized clinical trial.** *J Manipulative Physiol Ther.* March–April 1995;18(3):148–54.

101. Oliphant D. **Safety of spinal manipulation in the treatment of lumbar disk herniations: a systematic review and risk assessment.** *J Manipulative Physiol Ther.* March–April 2004;27(3):197–210. Review.

102. Rogers CM, Triano JJ. **Biomechanical measure validation for spinal manipulation in clinical settings.** *J Manipulative Physiol Ther.* November–December 2003;26(9):539–48.

103. Giles LG, Muller R. **Chronic spinal pain: a randomized clinical trial comparing medication, acupuncture, and spinal manipulation.** *Spine* (Phila Pa 1976). July 15, 2003;28(14):1490–1502; discussion 1502–3.

104. Hawk C, et al. **Feasibility study of short-term effects of chiropractic manipulation on older adults with impaired balance.** *J Chiropr Med.* December 2007;6(4):121–31.

105. Bove G, Nilsson N. **Spinal manipulation in the treatment of episodic tension-type headache: a randomized controlled trial.** *JAMA.* November 11, 1998;280(18):1576–79.

106. Bolton PS, Budgell BS. **Spinal manipulation and spinal mobilization influence different axial sensory beds.** *Med Hypotheses.* 2006;66(2):258–62.

107. Stuber KJ, Smith DL. **Chiropractic treatment of pregnancy-related low back pain: a systematic review of the evidence.** *J Manipulative Physiol Ther.* July–August 2008;31(6):447–54.

108. Nilsson N, Christensen HW, Hartvigsen J. **The effect of spinal manipulation in the treatment of cervicogenic headache.** *J Manipulative Physiol Ther.* June 1997;20(5):326–30.

109. Langenfeld A, et al. **Prognostic Factors for Recurrences in Neck Pain Patients Up to 1 Year After Chiropractic Care.** *J Manipulative Physiol Ther.* September 2015;38(7):458–64.

110. Hestbaek L, et al. **Low back pain in primary care: a description of 1,250 patients with low back pain in Danish general and chiropractic practice.** *Int J Family Med.* 2014;2014:106102.

111. Seaman DR, Palombo AD. **An overview of the identification and management of the metabolic syndrome in chiropractic practice.** *J Chiropr Med.* September 2014;13(3):210–19.

112. Goto V, et al. **Chiropractic intervention in the treatment of postmenopausal climacteric symptoms and insomnia:** A review. *Maturitas.* May 2014;78(1):3–7.

113. Sherrod C, Johnson D, Chester B. **Safety, tolerability and effectiveness of an ergonomic intervention with chiropractic care for knowledge workers with upper-extremity musculoskeletal disorders: a prospective case series.** *Work.* 2014;49(4):641–51.

114. Walker BF, et al. **Outcomes of usual chiropractic. The OUCH randomized controlled trial of adverse events.** *Spine* (Phila Pa 1976). September 15, 2013;38(20):1723–29.

115. Alcantara J, Alcantara JD, Alcantara J. **The chiropractic care of patients with cancer: a systematic review of the literature.** *Integr Cancer Ther.* December 2012;11(4):304–12.

116. Thorman P, Dixner A, Sundberg T. **Effects of chiropractic care on pain and function in patients with hip osteoarthritis waiting for arthroplasty: a clinical pilot trial.** *J Manipulative Physiol Ther.* July–August 2010;33(6):438–44.

117. Zhang J, Snyder BJ, Vernor L. **The effect of low force chiropractic adjustments on body surface electromagnetic field.** *J Can Chiropr Assoc.* March 2004;48(1):29–35.

118. Alcantara J, Ohm J, Kunz D. **The chiropractic care of children.** *J Altern Complement Med.* June 2010;16(6):621–26.

119. Shaw L, et al. **A systematic review of chiropractic management of adults with Whiplash-Associated Disorders: recommendations for advancing evidence-based practice and research.** *Work.* 2010;35(3):369–94.

120. Van Poecke AJ, Cunliffe C. **Chiropractic treatment for primary nocturnal enuresis: a case series of 33 consecutive patients.** *J Manipulative Physiol Ther.* October 2009;32(8):675–81.

121. Welch A, Boone R. **Sympathetic and parasympathetic responses to specific diversified adjustments to chiropractic vertebral subluxations of the cervical and thoracic spine.** *J Chiropr Med.* September 2008;7(3):86–93.

122. Christensen KD, Buswell K. **Chiropractic outcomes managing radiculopathy in a hospital setting: a retrospective review of 162 patients.** *J Chiropr Med.* September 2008;7(3):115–25.

123. Sandell J, Palmgren PJ, Björndahl L. **Effect of chiropractic treatment on hip extension ability and running velocity among young male running athletes.** *J Chiropr Med.* June 2008;7(2):39–47.
124. Borggren CL. **Pregnancy and chiropractic: a narrative review of the literature.** *J Chiropr Med.* June 2007;6(2):70–74.
125. Hoskins W, et al. **Chiropractic treatment of lower extremity conditions: a literature review.** *J Manipulative Physiol Ther.* October 2006;29(8):658–71. Review.
126. Smith DL, Dainoff MJ, Smith JP. **The effect of chiropractic adjustments on movement time: a pilot study using Fitts Law.** *J Manipulative Physiol Ther.* May 2006;29(4):257–66.
127. Dimmick KR, Young MF, Newell D. **Chiropractic manipulation affects the difference between arterial systolic blood pressures on the left and right in normotensive subjects.** *J Manipulative Physiol Ther.* January 2006;29(1):46.

Chapter 8: The Internet, Blood Pressure, and Emotions

1. Valderrama AL, et al. **Vital signs: Awareness and treatment of uncontrolled hypertension among adults—United States, 2003–2010.** Centers for Disease Control and Prevention: Morbidity and Mortality Weekly Report. September 7, 2012;61(35);703–9. http://www.cdc.gov/mmwr/preview/mmwrhtml/mm6135a3.htm.
2. Go AS, et al. **Heart disease and stroke statistics—2013 update: A report from the American Heart Association.** *Circulation.* 2013;127:e6–e245.
3. World Health Organization. ***Global health risks: mortality and burden of disease attributable to selected major risk.*** Geneva, Switzerland: WHO Press; 2009.
4. Ohkubo T, et al. **How many times should blood pressure be measured at home for better prediction of stroke risk? Ten-year follow-up results from the Ohasama study.** *J Hypertens.* June 2004;22(6):1099–104.
5. Muller DN, et al. **Immune-related effects in hypertension and target-organ damage.** *Current Opin Nephrol Hypertens.* March 2011;20(2):113–17.
6. Hermida RC, et al. **Around-the-clock ambulatory blood pressure monitoring is required to properly diagnose resistant hypertension and assess associated vascular risk.** *Curr Hypertens Rep.* July 2014;16(7):445.
7. Houston M. ***What Your Doctor May Not Tell You About Hypertension: The Revolutionary Nutrition and Lifestyle Program to Help Fight High Blood Pressure.*** New York, NY: Hachette Book Group; 2003.
8. Bonetti PO, et al. **Noninvasive identification of patients with early coronary atherosclerosis by assessment of digital reactive hyperemia.** *J Am Coll Cardiol.* 2004;44(11):2137–41.
9. Niiranen TJ, et al. **Office, home, and ambulatory blood pressures as predictors of cardiovascular risk.** *J Hypertension.* May 2014. pii: HYPERTENSIONAHA.114.03292. (Epub ahead of print.)
10. Rock W, et al. **The association between ambulatory systolic blood pressure and cardiovascular events in a selected population with intensive control of cardiovascular risk factors.** *J Am Soc Hypertens.* April 4, 2014. pii: S1933-1711(14)00448-3.

Chapter 9: The Pressure's On

1. Lopez MJ, et al. **Salt-resistant hypertension in mice lacking the guanylyl cyclase-A receptor for atrial natriuretic peptide.** *Nature.* November 1995;378(6552):65–68.
2. Weinberger, MH. **Salt sensitivity of blood pressure in humans.** *Hypertension.* 1996;27:481–90.
3. **Could low salt intake increase mortality risk?** *Medical News Today.* September 10, 2013. http://www.medicalnewstoday.com/articles/265814.php.
4. Horikawa C, et al. **Dietary sodium intake and incidence of diabetes complications in Japanese patients with type 2 diabetes: Analysis of the Japan Diabetes Complications Study (JDCS).** *Journal of Clinical Endocrinology & Metabolism.* July 22, 2014. http://press.endocrine.org/doi/abs/10.1210/jc.2013-4315?journalCode=jcem.
5. Schmidlin O, et al. **Chloride-dominant salt sensitivity in the stroke-prone spontaneously hypertensive rat.** *Hypertension.* May 2005;45:867–73.
6. McCallum L, et al. **Serum chloride is an independent predictor of mortality in hypertensive patients.** *Hypertension.* November 2013;62(5):836–43.
7. Wood, S. **Populationwide sodium guidance "makes no sense" in most countries.** *Medscape.* http://www.medscape.com/viewarticle/810431. September 4, 2013.
8. Kotchen, TA. **Contributions of Sodium and Chloride to NaCl-Induced Hypertension.** *Hypertension.* 2005;45:867–73.
9. Watson SE, et al. **Abstract 36: Adult hypertension risk is more than quadrupled in obese children.** *Hypertension.*

2013;62:836–43.

10. Whitescarver SA, et al. **Salt-sensitive hypertension: contribution of chloride.** *Science*. March 30, 1984;223(4643):1430–32.
11. Luft FC, et al. **Sodium bicarbonate and sodium chloride: effects on blood pressure and electrolyte homeostasis in normal and hypertensive man.** *J Hypertens*. July 1990;8(7):663–70.
12. Mahajan A, et al. **Daily oral sodium bicarbonate preserves glomerular filtration rate by slowing its decline in early hypertensive nephropathy.** *Kidney Int*. 2010;78(3):303–9.
13. Goraya N, et al. **A comparison of treating metabolic acidosis in CKD stage 4 hypertensive kidney disease with fruits and vegetables or sodium bicarbonate.** *Clin J Am Soc Nephrol*. March 2013;8(3):371–81.
14. Susantitaphong P, et al. **Short- and long-term effects of alkali therapy in chronic kidney disease: a systematic review.** *Am J Nephrol*. 2012;35(6):540–47.
15. Schmidlin O, et al. **Chloride-dominant salt sensitivity in the stroke-prone spontaneously hypertensive rat.** *Hypertension*. May 2005;45:867–73.
16. McCallum L, et al. **Serum chloride is an independent predictor of mortality in hypertensive patients.** *Hypertension*. November 2013;62(5):836–43.178. Kotchen, TA. **Contributions of Sodium and Chloride to NaCl-Induced Hypertension.** *Hypertension*. 2005;45:867–73.
17. Whitescarver SA, et al. **Salt-sensitive hypertension: contribution of chloride.** *Science*. March 30, 1984;223(4643):1430–32.
18. Luft FC, et al. **Sodium bicarbonate and sodium chloride: effects on blood pressure and electrolyte homeostasis in normal and hypertensive man.** *J Hypertens*. July 1990;8(7):663–70. 190. Schmidlin O, et al. **Chloride-dominant salt sensitivity in the stroke-prone spontaneously hypertensive rat.** *Hypertension*. May 2005;45:867–73.
19. McCallum L, et al. **Serum chloride is an independent predictor of mortality in hypertensive patients.** *Hypertension*. November 2013;62(5):836–43.
20. Kotchen, TA. **Contributions of sodium and chloride to NaCl-induced hypertension.** *Hypertension*. 2005;45:867–73.
21. Whitescarver SA, et al. **Salt-sensitive hypertension: contribution of chloride.** *Science*. March 30, 1984;223(4643):1430–32.
22. Luft FC, et al. **Sodium bicarbonate and sodium chloride: effects on blood pressure and electrolyte homeostasis in normal and hypertensive man.** *J Hypertens*. July 1990;8(7):663–70.
23. Yokoyama Y, et al. **Vegetarian diets and blood pressure.** *JAMA Internal Medicine*, 2014.
24. Haddy FJ, et al. **Role of potassium in regulating blood flow and blood pressure.** *Am J Physiol Regul Integr Comp Physiol*. March 2006;290(3):R546–52.
25. Sudhir K, et al. **Reduced dietary potassium reversibly enhances vasopressor response to stress in African Americans.** *Hypertension*. May 1997;29(5):1083–90.
26. Haddy FJ, et al. **Role of potassium in regulating blood flow and blood pressure.** *Am J Physiol Regul Integr Comp Physiol*. March 2006;290(3):R546–52.
27. **Neurogenic hypertension: Is the enigma of its origin near the solution?** *Hypertension*. 2004;43:154–55. Orig. pub. online December 15, 2003.
28. Ibid.
29. Eric Lazartigues. **Inflammation and neurogenic hypertension: A new role for the circumventricular organs?** Editorial. *Circulation Research*. 2010;107:166–67.
30. Wu KL, Chan SH, Chan JY. **Neuroinflammation and oxidative stress in rostral ventrolateral medulla contribute to neurogenic hypertension induced by systemic inflammation.** *J Neuroinflammation*. September 7, 2012;9(1):212.
31. Bakris G, et al. **Atlas vertebra realignment and achievement of arterial pressure goal in hypertensive patients: a pilot study.** *J Human Hypertens*. May 2007;21(5):347–52.
32. **Hyperthyroidism.** National Institutes of Health: MedlinePlus. http://www.nlm.nih.gov/medlineplus/ency/article/000356.htm. Updated June 7, 2013.
33. Oparil S, Sripairojthikoon W, Wyss JM. **The renal afferent nerves in the pathogenesis of hypertension.** *Can J Physiol Pharmacol*. August 1987;65(8):1548–58.
34. Nanba K, et al. **A subtype prediction score for primary aldosteronism.** *J Hum Hypertens*. Online publication April 3, 2014.
35. Alderman MH, et al. **Pressor responses to antihypertensive drug types.** *Am J Hypertens*. September 2010;23(9):1031–37.
36. Furberg CD. **Renin-guided treatment of hypertension: time for action.** *Am J Hypertens*. September 2010;23(9):929–30.
37. Ginty AT, et al. **Depression and anxiety are associated with a diagnosis of hypertension 5 years later in a cohort of late**

middle-aged men and women. *J Hum Hypertens.* March 2013;27(3):187–90.

38. Paz García-Vera M, et al. **Differences in emotional personality traits and stress between sustained hypertension and normotension.** *Hypertension Research.* March 2010;33:203–8.
39. Mayo Clinic Staff. **High blood pressure (hypertension): Medications and supplements that can raise your blood pressure.** Mayo Clinic. May 13, 2013. http://www.Mayoclinic.org/diseases-conditions/high-blood-pressure/in-depth/blood-pressure/art-20045245.
40. University of Pennsylvania School of Medicine. **Drinking alcohol provides no heart health benefit, new study shows.** ScienceDaily. July 10, 2014. http://www.sciencedaily.com/releases/2014/07/140710151947.htm.
41. Mayo Clinic Staff. **High blood pressure (hypertension): Medications and supplements that can raise your blood pressure.** Mayo Clinic. May 13, 2013. http://www.Mayoclinic.org/diseases-conditions/high-blood-pressure/in-depth/blood-pressure/art-20045245.
42. Mayo Clinic Staff. **High blood pressure (hypertension): Alternative medicine.** Mayo Clinic. April 28, 2014. http://www.Mayoclinic.org/diseases-conditions/high-blood-pressure/basics/alternative-medicine/con-20019580.
43. Sheps S. **High blood pressure (hypertension): Can L-arginine supplements lower blood pressure?** Mayo Clinic. April 2, 2014. http://www.Mayoclinic.org/diseases-conditions/high-blood-pressure/expert-answers/l-arginine/faq-20058052.
44. Rodríguez-Moran M, Guerrero-Romero F. **Oral magnesium supplementation improves the metabolic profile of metabolically obese, normal-weight individuals: a randomized double-blind placebo-controlled trial.** *Arch Med Res.* May 2014; pii: S0188-4409(14)00078-2.
45. Panhwar AH, et al. **Distribution of potassium, calcium, magnesium, and sodium levels in biological samples of Pakistani hypertensive patients and control subjects.** *Clin Lab.* 2014;60(3):463–74.
46. Houston M. **The role of nutrition and nutraceutical supplements in the treatment of hypertension.** *World J Cardiol.* February 26, 2014;6(2):38–66.
47. Yokoyama Y, et al. **Vegetarian diets and blood pressure: A meta analysis.** *JAMA Intern Med.* April 2014;174(4):577–87.
48. Jennings A, et al. **Amino Acid Intakes Are Inversely Associated with Arterial Stiffness and Central Blood Pressure in Women.** *J Nutr.* September 2015;145(9):2130–38.
49. Hughes JW, et al. **Randomized controlled trial of mindfulness-based stress reduction for prehypertension.** *Psychosomatic Medicine.* October 2013;75(8):721–28.
50. Cumming DC, Quigley ME, Yen SS. **Acute suppression of circulating testosterone levels by cortisol in men.** *J Clin Endocrinol Metab.* September 1983;57(3):671–73.
51. Alabdulgader AA. **Coherence: A Novel Nonpharmacological Modality for Lowering Blood Pressure in Hypertensive Patients.** *Global Advances in Health and Medicine.* May 2012;1(2):56–64.
52. Opendak M, Gould E. **Adult neurogenesis: a substrate for experience-dependent change.** *Trends in Cognitive Sciences,* 2015.
53. Rosanoff A, Weaver CM, Rude RK. **Suboptimal magnesium status in the United States: are the health consequences underestimated?** *Nutr Rev.* 2012, Mar;70(3):153–64.
54. Heath DL, Vink R. **Traumatic brain axonal injury in animals produced sustained decline in intracellular free magnesium concentration.** *Brain Res.* 1996;738:150–3.
55. Blaylock RL, Maroon J. **Natural plant products and extracts that reduce immunoexcitotoxicity-associated neurodegeneration and promote repair within the central nervous system.** *Surg Neurol Int.* 2012;3:19.
56. Rosanoff A, Weaver CM, Rude RK. **Suboptimal magnesium status in the United States: are the health consequences underestimated?** *Nutr Rev.* 2012, Mar;70(3):153–64.
57. Nielsen FH. **Effects of magnesium depletion on inflammation in chronic disease.** *Curr Opin Clin Nutr Metab Care.* 2014 Nov;17(6):525–30.
58. He K, et al. **Magnesium intake and incidence of metabolic syndrome among young adults.** *Circulation.* 2006;113(13):1675–82.
59. Chandrasekaran NC, et al. **Effects of magnesium deficiency—more than skin deep.** *Exp Biol Med* (Maywood). October 2014;239(10):1280–91.
60. Mauskop A, Varughese J. **Why all migraine patients should be treated with magnesium.** *J Neural Transm.* May 2012;119(5):575–79.
61. Nielsen FH. **Effects of magnesium depletion on inflammation in chronic disease.** *Curr Opin Clin Nutr Metab Care.* 2014

Nov;17(6):525–30.

62. Goldhamer AC, et al. **Medically supervised water-only fasting in the treatment of hypertension.** *J Manipulative Physiol Ther*. June 2001;24(5)335–39.
63. Goldhamer AC, et al. **Medically supervised water-only fasting in the treatment of borderline hypertension.** *J Altern Complement Med*. October 2002;8(5):643–50.
64. Valderrama AL, et al. **Vital signs: Awareness and treatment of uncontrolled hypertension among adults—United States, 2003–2010.** Centers for Disease Control and Prevention: Morbidity and Mortality Weekly Report. September 7, 2012;61(35):703–9. http://www.cdc.gov/mmwr/preview/mmwrhtml/mm6135a3.htm.
65. Go AS, et al. **Heart disease and stroke statistics—2013 update: a report from the American Heart Association.** *Circulation*. 2013;127:e6–e245.
66. **Vital signs: Awareness and treatment of uncontrolled hypertension among adults—United States, 2003–2010.** Centers for Disease Control and Prevention: Morbidity and Mortality Weekly Report. September 7, 2012;61(35):703–9. http://www.cdc.gov/mmwr/preview/mmwrhtml/mm6135a3.htm.
67. Gillum RF, Makuc DM, Feldman JJ. **Pulse rate, coronary heart disease, and death: the NHANES I epidemiologic follow-up study.** *Am Heart J*. January 1991;121(1 Pt 1):172–77.
68. Gillman MW, et al. **Influence of heart rate on mortality among persons with hypertension: The Framingham Study.** *Am Heart J*. April 1993;125(4):1148–54.
69. Fox K, et al. **Resting heart rate in cardiovascular disease.** *J Am Coll Cardiol*. August 28, 2007;50(9):823–30.
70. Cooney MT, et al. **Elevated resting heart rate is an independent risk factor for cardiovascular disease in healthy men and women.** *Am Heart J*. April 2010;159(4):612–19.
71. Ibid.
72. Hulbert AH. **Life and Death: Metabolic Rate, Membrane Composition, and Life Span of Animals.** *Physiological Reviews*. October 2007;87(4):1175–1213. http://physrev.physiology.org/content/87/4/1175.
73. Olshansky, SJ. **What Determines Longevity: Metabolic Rate or Stability?** July 25, 2009. Discovery Medicine. http://www.discoverymedicine.com/S-J-Olshansky/2009/07/25/what-determines-longevity-metabolic-rate-or-stability/.
74. Aguilaniu H, Durieux J, Dillin A. **Metabolism, ubiquinone synthesis, and longevity.** May 15, 2014. Genesdev.cshlp.org.
75. Walker TB, Robergs RA. **Does Rhodiola rosea possess ergogenic properties?** *International Journal of Sport Nutrition and Exercise Metabolism*. 2006;16(3):305.
76. Zhang Z, et al. **The effect of Rhodiola capsules on oxygen consumption of myocardium and coronary artery blood flow in dogs.** *Zhongguo Zhong Yao Za Zhi*. February 1998;23(2):104–6, inside back cover. Chinese.
77. Harris WS, et al. **Omega-3 fatty acids and coronary heart disease risk: clinical and mechanistic perspectives.** *Atherosclerosis*. March 2008;197(1):12–24.
78. Roffers SD, et al. **A somatovisceral reflex of lowered blood pressure and pulse rate after spinal manipulative therapy in the thoracic region.** *Asian J Multidiscipl Studies*. June 2015;3(6).
79. Budgell B, Hirano F. **Innocuous mechanical stimulation of the neck and alterations in heart-rate variability in healthy young adults.** *Auton Neurosci*. August 13, 2001;91(1–2):96–99.
80. Morrison RL, Bellack AS. **The role of social perception in social skill.** *Behavior Therapy*. January 1981;12(1):69–79.
81. Consoli SM, et al. **Differences in emotion processing in patients with essential and secondary hypertension.** *Am J Hypertens*. May 2010;23(5):515–21.
82. Baer PE, et al. **Behavioral response to induced conflict in families with a hypertensive father.** *Hypertension*. July-August 1980;2(4 Pt 2):70–77.

Chapter 10: Everything Is Connected, Everything Matters

1. Pert CB. ***Molecules of Emotion: The Science Behind Mind-Body Medicine.*** New York, NY: Simon & Schuster; 1999.

Chapter 11: It Takes a Village

1. Irimia A, Van Horn JD. **Systematic network lesioning reveals the core white matter scaffold of the human brain.** *Front Hum Neurosci*. February 11, 2014;8:51.
2. Getting PA. **Emerging principles governing the operation of neural networks.** *Ann Rev Neurosci*. March 1989;12:185–204.

3. Sporns O, et al. **Organization, development and function of complex brain networks.** *Trends in Cognitive Sciences*. September 2004;8(9):418–25.
4. Chatonnet F, Flamant F, Morte B. **A temporary compendium of thyroid hormone target genes in brain.** *Biochim Biophys Acta*. May 31, 2014.
5. Remaud S, et al. **Thyroid hormone signaling and adult neurogenesis in mammals.** *Front Endocrinol* (Lausanne). April 28, 2014;5:62.
6. Schroeder AC, Privalsky ML. **Thyroid hormones, t3 and t4, in the brain.** *Front Endocrinol* (Lausanne). March 31, 2014;5:40.
7. Splendiani A, et al. **Magnetic resonance imaging (MRI) of the lumbar spine with dedicated G-scan machine in the upright position: a retrospective study and our experience in 10 years with 4305 patients.** *Radiol Med*. July 28, 2015. (Epub ahead of print.) PubMed PMID: 26215713.
8. Ibid.
9. Knudsen N, et al. **Small differences in thyroid function may be important for body mass index and the occurrence of obesity in the population.** *Journal of Clinical Endocrinology & Metabolism*. July 1, 2005;90(7):4019–24.
10. Moulin de Moraes CM, et al. **Prevalence of subclinical hypothyroidism in a morbidly obese population and improvement after weight loss induced by Roux-en-Y gastric bypass.** *Obes Surg*. 2005 Oct;15(9):1287–91.

Chapter 12: That Little Gland Does What?

1. Walter, KN, et al. **Elevated thyroid stimulating hormone is associated with elevated cortisol in healthy young men and women.** *Thyroid Research*. October 30, 2012;5(1):13.
2. Karthick N, et al. **Dyslipidaemic changes in women with subclinical hypothyroidism.** *J Clin Diagn Res*. October 2013;7(10):2122–25.
3. Ibid.
4. Moseley KF. **Type 2 diabetes and bone fractures.** *Curr Opin Endocrinol Diabetes Obes*. April 2012;19(2):128–35.
5. Van den Beld AW, et al. **Thyroid hormone concentrations, disease, physical function, and mortality in elderly men.** *Journal of Clinical Endocrinology & Metabolism*. December 2005;90(12):6403–9.
6. Holtorf K. **Thyroid Hormone Transport into Cellular Tissue.** *Journal of Restorative Medicine*. April 2014;3(4):53–68.
7. Van den Beld AW, et al. **Thyroid hormone concentrations, disease, physical function, and mortality in elderly men.** *Journal of Clinical Endocrinology & Metabolism*. December 2005;90(12):6403–9.
8. Fraser WD, et al. **Are biochemical tests of thyroid function of any value in monitoring patients receiving thyroxine replacement?** *BMJ*. 1986;293:808–10.
9. Bochukova E, et al. **A mutation in the thyroid hormone receptor alpha gene.** *N Engl J Med*. 2012;366:243–49.
10. Alevizaki M, et al. **TSH may not be a good marker for adequate thyroid hormone replacement therapy.** *Wien Klin Wochenschr*. 2005;117(18):636–40.
11. Holtorf K. **Thyroid Hormone Transport into Cellular Tissue.** *Journal of Restorative Medicine*. April 2014;3(4):53–68.1.
12. Ibid.
13. Van den Beld AW, et al. **Thyroid hormone concentrations, disease, physical function, and mortality in elderly men.** *Journal of Clinical Endocrinology & Metabolism*. December 2005;90(12):6403–9.
14. Fraser WD, et al. **Are biochemical tests of thyroid function of any value in monitoring patients receiving thyroxine replacement?** *BMJ*. 1986;293:808–10.
15. Escobar-Morreale HF, et al. **Replacement therapy for hypothyroidism with thyroxine alone does not ensure euthyroidism in all tissues, as studied in thyroidectomized rats.** *J Clin Invest*. 1995;96(6):2828–38.
16. Engbring N, Engstrom W. **Effects of estrogen and testosterone on circulating thyroid hormone.** *J Clin Endocrinol Metab*. July 1, 1959;19(7):783–96.
17. Wilber JF, Utiger RD. **The effect of glucocorticoids on thyrotropin secretion.** *J Clin Invest*. November 1969;48(11):2096–2103.
18. Blackwell J. **Evaluation and treatment of hyperthyroidism and hypothyroidism.** *J Am Acad Nurse Pract*. October 2004;16(10):422–25.
19. Maruo T, et al. **A role for thyroid hormone in the induction of ovulation and corpus luteum function.** *Horm Res*. 1992;37(Suppl 1):12–18.
20. De Lean A, et al. **Modulation of pituitary thyrotropin releasing hormone receptor levels by estrogens and thyroid**

hormones. *Endocrinology*. June 1, 1977;100(6).

Chapter 13: Problems with Smoothies?

1. Ledesma L, et al. **Monounsaturated fatty acid (avocado) rich diet for mild hypercholesterolemia.** *Arch-Med-Res*. Winter 1996;27(4): 519–23.
2. Wang L, et al. **Effect of a Moderate Fat Diet With and Without Avocados on Lipoprotein Particle Number, Size and Subclasses in Overweight and Obese Adults: A Randomized, Controlled Trial.** *J Am Heart Assoc*. 2015;4(1):e001355.

Chapter 14: Are Your Symptoms Really Consequences?

1. Clementson CE, et al. **Inflammation is detrimental for neurogenesis in adult brain.** *Proc Natl Acad Sci USA*. November 11, 2003;100(23):13632-13637.
2. Cohen IR, et al., eds. ***Advances in Experimental Medicine and Biology***. New York, NY: Springer Science + Business Media; 1976: 517–27.
3. Lopez-Ramirez MA, Wu D, Pryce G, et al. **MicroRNA-155 negatively affects blood-brain barrier function during neuroinflammation.** *FASEB J*. June 2014;28(6):2551–65.
4. Destefano M. **Ego city: Cities are organized like human brains.** *ScienceDaily*. September 19, 2009. http://www.sciencedaily.com/releases/2009/09/090903163945.htm.

Chapter 15: Seeds of Health

1. Kwan CL, et al. **Abnormal forebrain activity in functional bowel disorder patients with chronic pain.** *Neurology*, October 25, 2005;65(8):1268–77.
2. Meerman EE, Verkuil B, Brosschot JF. **Decreasing pain tolerance outside of awareness.** *J Psychosom Res*. March 2001;70(3):250–57.
3. McDougall JJ. **Arthritis and pain. Neurogenic origin of joint pain.** *Arthritis Res Ther*. 2006;8(6):220.
4. Walton KD, Dubois M, Linas RR. **Abnormal thalamocortical activity in patients with complex regional pain syndrome (CRPS) type I.** *Pain*. July 2010;150(1):41–51.
5. Schulze J, Troeger C. **Increased sympathetic activity assessed by special analysis of heart rate variability in patients with CRPS I.** *Handchir Mikrochir Plast Chir*. February 2010;42(1):44–48.
6. Montalto M, et al. **Fructose, trehalose and sorbitol malabsorption.** *Eur Rev Med Pharmacol Sci*. 2013;17 Suppl 2:26–29.
7. Elphick HL, Elphick DA, Sanders DS. **Small bowel bacterial overgrowth. An underrecognized cause of malnutrition in older adults.** *Geriatrics*. September 2006;61(9):21–26.
8. Dukowicz AC, Lacy BE, Levine GM. **Small intestinal bacterial overgrowth: a comprehensive review.** *Gastroenterology Hepatol (NY)*. February 2007;3(2):112–22.
9. Gabrielli M, et al. **Prevalence of Small Intestinal Bacterial Overgrowth in Parkinson's Disease.** *Mov. Disord*. 2011;26:889–92.
10. Biesiekierski JR, et al. **No Effects of Gluten in Patients With Self-Reported Non-Celiac Gluten Sensitivity After Dietary Reduction of Fermentable, Poorly Absorbed, Short-Chain Carbohydrates.** *Gastroenterology*. 2013;145:320–28.
11. Halmos EP, et al. **A Diet Low in FODMAPs Reduces Symptoms of Irritable Bowel Syndrome.** *Gastroenterology*. 146(1):67–75.e5.
12. Staudacher, HM, et al. **Comparison of symptom response following advice for a diet low in fermentable carbohydrates (FODMAPs) versus standard dietary advice in patients with irritable bowel syndrome.** *Journal of Human Nutrition and Dietetics*. 2011;24:487–495.
13. Stefka AT, et al. **Commensal bacteria protect against food allergen sensitization.** *Proceedings of the National Academy of Sciences*. September 9, 2014;111(36):13145–50. (Published online August 25, 2014.)
14. Kostic, AD, et al. **The Dynamics of the Human Infant Gut Microbiome in Development and in Progression toward Type 1 Diabetes.** *Cell Host & Microbe*. February 11, 2015;17(2):260–73.
15. Ibid.
16. Ibid.
17. Qiao Y, et al. **Effects of resveratrol on gut microbiota and fat storage in a mouse model with high-fat-induced obesity.** *Food Funct*. June 28, 2014;5(6):1241–49.
18. Schnabl B, Brenner DA. **Interactions between the intestinal microbiome and liver diseases.** *Gastroenterology*. May

2014;146(6):1513–24.
19. Eaton K, et al. **Abnormal gut fermentation: Laboratory studies reveal deficiency of B vitamins, zinc, and magnesium.** *Journal of Nutritional Biochemistry*. November 1993;4(11):635–38.
20. Henao-Mejia J, Elinav E, Jin C. **Inflammasome-mediated dysbiosis regulates progression of NAFLD and obesity.** *Nature*. February 9, 2012;482:179–85.
21. Amar J, et al. **Intestinal mucosal adherence and translocation of commensal bacteria at the early onset of type 2 diabetes: Molecular mechanisms and probiotic treatment.** *EMBO Mol Med*. September 2011;3(9):559–72.
22. Iannitti T, Palmieri B. **Therapeutical use of probiotic formulations in clinical practice.** *Clinical Nutrition*. December 2010;29(6):701–25.
23. Brewer GJ. **Copper excess, zinc deficiency, and cognition loss in Alzheimer's disease.** *Biofactors*. 2012;38:107–13.
24. Watt NT, Whitehouse IJ, Hooper NM. **The role of zinc in Alzheimer's disease.** *Int J Alzheimer's Dis*. 2011;2011:971021.
25. Moon C, et al. **Vertically transmitted faecal IgA levels determine extra-chromosomal phenotypic variation.** *Nature*. 2015.
26. Ryan KK, et al. **FXR is a molecular target for the effects of vertical sleeve gastrectomy.** *Nature*. May 8, 2014;509:183–88.
27. Zeevi D, et al. **Personalized Nutrition by Prediction of Glycemic Responses.** *Cell*. 163(5):1079–94.
28. Grundy SM. **Pre-diabetes, metabolic syndrome, and cardiovascular risk.** *J Am Coll Cardiol*. February 14, 2012;59(7):635–43. doi: 10.1016/j.jacc.2011.08.080. Review.
29. Ibid.
30. Stanford University. **Low FODMAP Diet.** http://fodmapliving.com/the-science/stanford-university-low-fodmap-diet/.

Chapter 16: Wolves and the Big Picture

1. Abel R. ***The Eye Care Revolution: Prevent and Reverse Common Vision Problems.*** New York, NY: Kensington Books; 2004.
2. Liu Y, et al. **Liver-directed neonatal gene therapy prevents cardiac, bone, ear, and eye disease in mucopolysaccharidosis I mice.** *Mol Ther*. 2006;11:35–47.
3. O'Neill DP. **The eye and liver disorders.** *Eye*. 1992;6(4):366–70.
4. Müller A, Rehm WF, Vuilleumier JP. **Studies on the vitamin A level in the liver and serum of cattle in their relationship to the photography of the fundus of the eye.** *Zentralblatt für Veterinärmedizin*. August 1970;17(7):652–62.
5. Mehling WE, Krause N. **Are difficulties perceiving and expressing emotions associated with low-back pain? The relationship between lack of emotional awareness (alexithymia) and 12-month prevalence of low-back pain in 1180 urban public transit operators.** *J Psychosom Res*. January 2005;58(1):73–81.
6. Esteves JE, et al. **Emotional processing and its relationship to chronic low back pain: results from a case-control study.** *Man Ther*. December 2013;18(6):541–46.
7. Carson JW, et al. **Conflict about expressing emotions and chronic low back pain: associations with pain and anger.** *J Pain*. May 2007;8(5):405–11.
8. Middleton P, Pollard H. **Are chronic low back pain outcomes improved with co-management of concurrent depression?** *Chiropr Osteopat*. June 22, 2005;13(1):8.
9. Moore JE. **Chronic low back pain and psychosocial issues.** *Phys Med Rehabil Clin N Am*. November 2010;21(4):801–15.
10. Schofferman J, et al. **Childhood psychological trauma correlates with unsuccessful lumbar spine surgery.** *Spine* (Philadelphia, PA 1976). June 1992;17(6 Suppl):S138–44.
11. Klinghardt D. **Lehrbuch der Psycho-Kinesiologie.** Institut Für Neurobiologie. 12. Aufl., Juni 2013.
12. Schofferman J, et al. **Childhood psychological trauma and chronic refractory low-back pain.** *Clin J Pain*. December 1993;9(4):260–65.
13. Tzanoulinou S, et al. **Long-Term Behavioral Programming Induced by Peripuberty Stress in Rats Is Accompanied by GABAergic-Related Alterations in the Amygdala.** Schmidt MV, ed. *PLoS ONE*. 2014;9(4):e94666.
14. Marquez C, et al. **Peripuberty stress leads to abnormal aggression, altered amygdala and orbitofrontal reactivity and increased prefrontal MAOA gene expression.** *Transl Psychiatry*. 2013;3:e216.
15. Menga G, et al. **Fibromyalgia: Can Online Cognitive Behavioral Therapy Help?** *Ochsner Journal*. 2014;14(3):343–49.
16. Ibid.
17. Van Ballegooijen W, et al. **Adherence to Internet-Based and Face-to-Face Cognitive Behavioural Therapy for Depression: A Meta-Analysis.** García AV, ed. *PLoS ONE*. 2014;9(7):e100674.

18. Van Beugen S, et al. **Internet-Based Cognitive Behavioral Therapy for Patients With Chronic Somatic Conditions: A Meta-Analytic Review.** Eysenbach G, ed. *Journal of Medical Internet Research*. 2014;16(3):e88.
19. Lowes R. **Specialist office visits outpaced primary care in 2013.** Medscape. May 7, 2014. http://www.medscape.com/viewarticle/824733.
20. **A wolf's role in the ecosystem—the trophic cascade.** Mission: Wolf. http://www.missionwolf.org/page/trophic-cascade/.
21. Ripple, WJ, Beschta RL. **Trophic cascades in Yellowstone: The first 15 years after wolf reintroduction.** *Biol. Conserv.* January 2012;145(1):205–13.
22. Monbiot G. **For more wonder, rewild the world.** Talk presented at TED Global 2013. June 2013, Edinburgh, Scotland. http://www.ted.com/talks/george_monbiot_for_more_wonder_rewild_the_world.
23. Oregon State University News Research and Communications. **Of bears and berries: Return of wolves aids grizzly bears in Yellowstone.** Oregon State University. July 29, 2013. http://oregonstate.edu/ua/ncs/archives/2013/jul/bears-and-berries-return-wolves-aids-grizzly-bears-yellowstone.

Chapter 18: How to Make the Weight Slide Right Off

1. Corinna Noel, Robin Dando. **The effect of emotional state on taste perception.** *Appetite*. 2015.

Chapter 19: A Sick Dog's Weight-Loss Lessons

1. Allison DB, et al. **Annual deaths attributable to obesity in the United States.** *JAMA*. 1999;282:1530–38.
2. Chuang YF, et al. **Midlife adiposity predicts earlier onset of Alzheimer's dementia, neuropathology and presymptomatic cerebral amyloidaccumulation.** Mol Psychiatry. 2015 Sep 1. doi: 10.1038/mp.2015.129. (Epub ahead of print.) PubMed PMID: 26324099.
3. Ekelund U, et al. **Physical activity and all-cause mortality across levels of overall and abdominal adiposity in European men and women: The European Prospective Investigation into Cancer and Nutrition Study (EPIC).** *Am J Clin Nutr.* January 14, 2015.
4. Ng M, et al. **Global, regional, and national prevalence of overweight and obesity in children and adults during 1980–2013: A systematic analysis for the Global Burden of Disease Study 2013.** *Lancet*. May 28, 2014. pii: S0140-6736(14)60460-8.
5. Ford ES, Maynard LM, Li C. **Trends in Mean Waist Circumference and Abdominal Obesity Among US Adults, 1999–2012.** *JAMA*. 2014;312(11):1151–53.
6. Rawlings AM, et al. **Diabetes in midlife and cognitive change over 20 years: A cohort study.** *Ann Intern Med.* 2014;161:785–93).
7. **Type 2 Diabetes May Shrink the Brain.** WebMD: Diabetes Health Center. http://www.webmd.com/diabetes/news/20140429/type-2-diabetes-May-shrink-the-brain-study-suggests?src=RSS_PUBLIC.
8. Gregg EW, et al. **Trends in lifetime risk and years of life lost due to diabetes in the USA, 1985–2011: A modelling study.** *Lancet Diabetes & Endocrinology*. August 13, 2014.
9. Kolata G. **Looking Past Blood Sugar to Survive With Diabetes.** August 20, 2007. http://www.nytimes.com/2007/08/20/health/20diabetes.html?adxnnlx=1411225707-s8oNCsEcMoKAbxxleIdfog&pagewanted=all.
10. Diabetes Prevention Program Research Group. **10-year follow-up of diabetes incidence and weight loss, in the Diabetes Prevention Program Outcomes Study.** *Lancet.* November 14, 2009;374(9702):1677–86.
11. Basu S, et al. **The relationship of sugar to population-level diabetes prevalence: an econometric analysis of repeated cross-sectional data.** *PLoS One*. 2013;8:e57873.
12. Malhotra A, Noakes T, Phinney S. **It is time to bust the myth of physical inactivity and obesity: you cannot outrun a bad diet.** *Br J Sports Med.* April 22, 2015. pii: bjsports-2015-094911.
13. Feinman RD, et al. **Dietary carbohydrate restriction as the first approach in diabetes management: Critical review and evidence base.** *Nutrition*. January 2015;31(1):1–13.
14. St-Onge M, Janssen I, Heymsfield SB. **Metabolic Syndrome in Normal-Weight Americans: New definition of the metabolically obese, normal-weight individual.** *Diabetes Care*. September 2004;27(9):2222–28.
15. Weiss R, Bremer AA, Lustig RH. **What is metabolic syndrome, and why are children getting it?** *Ann NY Acad Sci.* April

2013;1281:123–40. Epub Jan 28, 2013. Review.
16. American Psychological Association. **Stress in America: Paying With Our Health.** February 4, 2015. http://www.apa.org/news/press/releases/stress/2014/stress-report.pdf.
17. Elia M. **Organ and tissue contribution to metabolic weight.** In: Kinney JM, Tucker HN, eds. ***Energy Metabolism: Tissue Determinants and Cellular Corollaries.*** New York, NY: Raven Press; 1992: 61–79.
18. Suez J, et al. **Artificial sweeteners induce glucose intolerance by altering the gut microbiota.** *Nature.* September 2014; 514(7521):181–86.
19. Fowler SPG, Williams K, Hazuda HP. **Diet Soda Intake Is Associated with Long-Term Increases in Waist Circumference in a Biethnic Cohort of Older Adults.** The San Antonio Longitudinal Study of Aging. *Journal of the American Geriatrics Society.* March 17, 2015.
20. Padayatty SJ, et al. **Human adrenal glands secrete vitamin C in response to adrenocorticotrophic hormone.** *Am J Clin Nutr.* July 2007;86(1):145–49.
21. Onge MP, et al. **Sleep restriction leads to increased activation of brain regions sensitive to food stimuli.** Institute of Human Nutrition, College of Physicians and Surgeons, Columbia University, New York, NY. *Am J Clin Nutr.* April 2012;95(4):818–24.

Chapter 20: Obesity and Inflammation: A Terrible Twosome

1. Simpson ER, Brown KA. **Obesity and breast cancer: a tale of inflammation and dysregulated metabolism.** *Mol Endocrinol.* May 2013;27(5):715–25. Review.
2. Kappelman MFD, et al. **The prevalence and geographic distribution of Crohn's disease and ulcerative colitis in the United States.** *Clin Gastroenterol Hepatol.* 2007;5:1424–29.
3. Wilcox CS, et al. **Repeated mixing and isolation: measuring chronic, intermittent stress in Holstein calves.** *J Dairy Sci,* Nov 2013;96(11):7223–33.
4. Allen LV, Jr. **Adrenal fatigue.** *Int J Pharm Compd.* Jan–Feb 2013;17(1):39–44.
5. Munsterhjelm K, et al. **Physicians defend Scandlab: Salivary cortisol test can determine adrenal fatigue.** *Lakartidningen.* May 25–31, 2011;108(21):1196–97; discussion 1197–98. Swedish.
6. Nippoldt T. Mayo Clinic office visit. **Adrenal fatigue. An interview with Todd Nippoldt, M.D.** *Mayo Clin Womens Healthsource.* March 2010;14(3):6.
7. Tome ME, McNabb FM, Gwazdauskas FC. **Adrenal responses to chronic and acute water stress in Japanese quail *Coturnix japonica.*** *Comp Biochem Physiol A Comp Physiol.* 1985;81(1):171–79.
8. Moss HB, et al. **Salivary cortisol responses in prepubertal boys: The effects of parental substance abuse and association with drug use behavior during adolescence.** *Biol Psychiatry.* May 15, 1999;45(10):1293–99.
9. Nieman LK. **Screening for reversible osteoporosis: Is cortisol a culprit?** *Ann Intern Med.* 2007;147(8):582–84.
10. Lupien SJ, et al. **Cortisol levels during human aging predict hippocampal atrophy and memory deficits.** *Nature Neuroscience* 1.1 (1998): 69–73.
11. Randall M. **The Physiology of Stress: Cortisol and the Hypothalamic-Pituitary-Adrenal Axis.** Dartmouth University. February 3, 2011. http://dujs.dartmouth.edu/fall-2010/the-physiology-of-stress-cortisol-and-the-hypothalamic-pituitary-adrenal-axis#.U5POyij5cuA.
12. Chrousos GP. **Stress and disorders of the stress system.** *Nature Reviews Endocrinology.* July 2009;5:374–81.
13. Lupien SJ, et al. **Cortisol levels during human aging predict hippocampal atrophy and memory deficits.** *Nature Neuroscience* 1.1 (1998): 69–73.
14. Randall M. **The Physiology of Stress: Cortisol and the Hypothalamic-Pituitary-Adrenal Axis.** Dartmouth University. February 3, 2011. http://dujs.dartmouth.edu/fall-2010/the-physiology-of-stress-cortisol-and-the-hypothalamic-pituitary-adrenal-axis#.U5POyij5cuA.
15. Chrousos GP. **Stress and disorders of the stress system.** *Nature Reviews Endocrinology.* July 2009;5:374–81.
16. Vauthier V, et al. **Endospanin 1 silencing in the hypothalamic arcuate nucleus contributes to sustained weight loss of high fat diet obese mice.** *Gene Ther.* July 2014;21(7):638–44.
17. Andrews R, Walker B. **Glucocorticoids and insulin resistance: old hormones, new targets.** *Clinical Science.* 1999;96(6):513–23.
18. Chen K, et al. **Induction of leptin resistance through direct interaction of C-reactive protein with leptin.** *Nature Medicine.* April 2006;12(4):425–32.

19. Carney DR, Cuddy AJ, Yap AJ. **Power posing: Brief nonverbal displays affect neuroendocrine levels and risk tolerance.** *Psychological Science.* 2010;21(10):1363–68.
20. Ibid.
21. Peper E, Lin, IM. **Increase or decrease depression: How body postures influence your energy level.** *Biofeedback.* 2012;40(3):126–30.
22. Cuddy A. **Boost Power Through Body Language.** HBR Blog Network. *Harvard Business Review.* April 6, 2011.
23. Youm Y-H, et al. **The ketone metabolite β-hydroxybutyrate blocks NLRP3 inflammasome–mediated inflammatory disease.** *Nature Medicine,* 2015;21(3):263–69.
24. Boyd DB. **Insulin and cancer.** *Integr Cancer Ther.* December 2003;2(4):315–29.
25. Ibid.
26. Björntorp P. **Metabolic implications of body fat distribution.** *Diabetes Care.* December 1991;14(12):1132–43.
27. Armougom F, et al. **Monitoring bacterial community of human gut microbiota reveals an increase in Lactobacillus in obese patients and Methanogens in anorexic patients.** *PLoS ONE* 4(9),e7125 (2009).
28. Raoult D. **Obesity pandemics and the modification of digestive bacterial flora.** *Eur. J. Clin. Microbiol. Infect. Dis.*27(8),631–34 (2008).
29. Gordon JI, Klaenhammer TR. **A rendezvous with our microbes.** *Proc. Natl Acad. Sci. USA* 108(Suppl. 1),S4513–S4515 (2011).
30. Khoruts A, Sadowsky MJ. **Therapeutic transplantation of the distal gut microbiota.** *Mucosal. Immunol.*4(1),4–7 (2011).
31. Raoult D. **Probiotics and obesity: a link?** *Nat. Rev. Microbiol.* 7,619 (2009).
32. Raoult D. **Human microbiome: take-home lesson on growth promoters?** *Nature* 454(7205),690–91 (2008).

Chapter 21: Your Hormones and Stress

1. Selye H. ***The Story of the Adaptation Syndrome.*** Montreal, Quebec: ACTA Inc.; 1952.
2. Selye H. ***The Stress of Life.*** New York, NY: McGraw-Hill; 1956.
3. Selye H. ***Stress without distress.*** Philadelphia, PA: J. B. Lippincott Co.; 1974.
4. Selye H. **Relation of the adrenal cortex to arthritis.** *Lancet.* June 22, 1946;247(6408):942.
5. Selye H. ***The Stress of Life.*** New York, NY: McGraw-Hill; 1956.
6. Selye H. ***Stress without distress.*** Philadelphia, PA: J. B. Lippincott Co.; 1974.
7. Selye H. ***The Stress of Life.*** New York, NY: McGraw-Hill; 1956.
8. Selye H. ***Stress without distress.*** Philadelphia, PA: J. B. Lippincott Co.; 1974.
9. Selye H. **Relation of the adrenal cortex to arthritis.** *Lancet.* June 22, 1946;247(6408):942.
10. Selye H. **Factors influencing the production of cardiovascular diseases by anterior pituitary and corticoid hormones.** *Endocrinology.* 1946;39:71.
11. Selye H. ***The Physiology and Pathology of Exposure to Stress: A Treatise Based on the Concepts of the General-Adaptation-Syndrome and the Diseases of Adaptation.*** Montreal, Quebec: ACTA Inc.; 1950.
12. Selye H. **Factors influencing the production of cardiovascular diseases by anterior pituitary and corticoid hormones.** *Endocrinology.* 1946;39:71.
13. Giltay EJ, et al. **Dispositional optimism and all-cause and cardiovascular mortality in a prospective cohort of elderly Dutch men and women.** *Arch Gen Psychiatry.* November 2004;61(11):1126–35.
14. Gallacher D, Gallacher J. **Are relationships good for your health?** *Student BMJ.* January 2011;19:d404.
15. King KB, Reis HT. **Marriage and long-term survival after coronary artery bypass grafting.** *Health Psychol.* January 2012;31(1):55–62.
16. Oliver KN, et al. **Stigma and optimism in adolescents and young adults with cystic fibrosis.** *J Cyst Fibros.* May 1, 2014. pii: S1569-1993(14)00092-7.
17. Popa-Velea O, Purcarea VL. **Psychological factors mediating health-related quality of life in COPD.** *J Med Life.* March 15, 2014;7(1):100–3.
18. Erlik Y, Meldrum DR, Judd HL. **Estrogen levels in postmenopausal women with hot flashes.** *Obstetrics & Gynecology.* April 1982;59(4):403–538.

19. Woods NF, et al. **Increased urinary cortisol levels during the menopausal transition.** *Menopause*. March–April 2006;13(2):212–21.
20. Food and Agriculture Organization of the United Nations: FAO Soils Bulletin 17: **Trace Elements in Soil and Agriculture.** 1972.
21. Thomas D. **The mineral depletion of foods available to us as a nation (1940–2002)—a review of the 6th Edition of McCance and Widdowson.** *Nutr Health*. 2007;19(1-2):21–55.
22. Tan ZX, Lal R, Wiebe KD. **Global soil nutrient depletion and yield reduction.** *J Sustain Agr*. 2005;26(1):123–46.
23. Pacifico D, et al. **NMR-based metabolomics for organic farming traceability of early potatoes.** *J Agric Food Chem*. November 20, 2013;61(46):11201–11.
24. Gordon B. **Manganese nutrition of glyphosate-resistant and conventional soybeans.** *Better Crops*. 2007;91(4):12–13.
25. Hunter D, et al. **Evaluation of the micronutrient composition of plant foods produced by organic and conventional agricultural methods.** *Crit Rev Food Sci Nutr*. July 2011;51(6):571–82. Review.
26. Györéné KG, Varga A, Lugasi A. **A comparison of chemical composition and nutritional value of organically and conventionally grown plant derived foods.** *Orv Hetil*. October 29, 2006;147(43):2081–90. Review.
27. Mahan DC, Peters JC. **Long-term effects of dietary organic and inorganic selenium sources and levels on reproducing sows and their progeny.** *J Anim Sci*. May 2004;82(5):1343–58.
28. Gordon B. **Manganese nutrition of glyphosate-resistant and conventional soybeans.** *Better Crops*. 2007;91(4):12–13.
29. Hunter D, et al. **Evaluation of the micronutrient composition of plant foods produced by organic and conventional agricultural methods.** *Crit Rev Food Sci Nutr*. July 2011;51(6):571–82. Review.
30. Györéné KG, Varga A, Lugasi A. **A comparison of chemical composition and nutritional value of organically and conventionally grown plant derived foods.** *Orv Hetil*. October 29, 2006;147(43):2081–90. Review.
31. Akbaba U, Sahin Y, Türkez H. **Element content analysis by WDXRF in pistachios grown under organic and conventional farming regimes for human nutrition and health.** *Toxicol Ind Health*. October 2012;28(9):783–38.
32. Vanzo A, et al. **Metabolomic profiling and sensorial quality of "Golden Delicious," "Liberty," "Santana," and "Topaz" apples grown using organic and integrated production systems.** *J Agric Food Chem*. July 3, 2013;61(26):6580–87.
33. Nitika, Punia D, Khetarpaul N. **Physico-chemical characteristics, nutrient composition and consumer acceptability of wheat varieties grown under organic and inorganic farming conditions.** *Int J Food Sci Nutr*. May 2008;59(3):224–45.
34. Gordon B. **Manganese nutrition of glyphosate-resistant and conventional soybeans.** *Better Crops*. 2007;91(4):12–13.
35. Hunter D, et al. Review: **Evaluation of the micronutrient composition of plant foods produced by organic and conventional agricultural methods.** *Crit Rev Food Sci Nutr*. July 2011;51(6):571–82.
36. Györéné KG, Varga A, Lugasi A. **A comparison of chemical composition and nutritional value of organically and conventionally grown plant derived foods.** *Orv Hetil*. October 29, 2006;147(43):2081–90. Review.
37. Akbaba U, Sahin Y, Türkez H. **Element content analysis by WDXRF in pistachios grown under organic and conventional farming regimes for human nutrition and health.** *Toxicol Ind Health*. October 2012;28(9):783–88.
38. Vanzo A, et al. **Metabolomic profiling and sensorial quality of "Golden Delicious," "Liberty," "Santana," and "Topaz" apples grown using organic and integrated production systems.** *J Agric Food Chem*. July 3, 2013;61(26):6580–87.
39. Chensheng Lu, et al. **Organic diets significantly lower children's dietary exposure to organophosphorus pesticides.** *Environ Health Perspect*. Feb 2006;114(2):260–63.
40. Repetto R, Baliga SS. **Pesticides and the Immune System: The Public Health Risks.** Executive summary. *Cent Eur J Public Health*. December 1996;4(4):263–65.
41. Obayashi Y, et al. ***Interdisciplinary Studies on Environmental Chemistry, Vol. 2: Environmental Research in Asia for Establishing a Scientist's Network.*** Tokyo: Terrapub; 2009: 211–17.
42. Colborn T, vom Saal FS, Soto AM. **Developmental effects of endocrine-disrupting chemicals in wildlife and humans.** *Environmental Health Perspectives*. 1993;101(5):378–84.
43. Bretveld RW, et al. **Pesticide exposure: The hormonal function of the female reproductive system disrupted?** *Reproductive Biology and Endocrinology*. 2006;4:30.
44. Eskenazi B, et al. **Prenatal exposure to pesticides can lead to problems with brain development in children. Pesticide toxicity and the developing brain.** *Basic Clin Pharmacol Toxicol*. February 2008;102(2):228–36.
45. Furlong CE, et al. **Children have higher cumulative rates of pesticides in their bodies. Newborns and children have a greater risk from pesticide exposure than adults. PON1 status of farmworker mothers and children as a predictor of organophosphate sensitivity.** *Pharmacogenet Genomics*. March 2006;16(3):183–90.

46. Landrigan PJ, et al. **Pesticides and inner-city children: Exposures, risks, and prevention.** *Environmental Health Perspectives* 1999;107(Suppl 3):431–37.
47. Garry V, et al. **Pesticide appliers, biocides, and birth defects in rural Minnesota.** *Environmental Health Perspectives.* 1996;104(4):394–99.
48. Salam MT, et al. **Early life environmental risk factors for asthma: Findings from the children's health study.** *Environmental Health Perspectives.* 2003;112(6):760.
49. Hernández AF, Parrón T, and Alarcón R. **Pesticides and asthma.** *Curr Opin Allergy Clin Immunol.* 2011;11(2):90–6.
50. Rui L, Haoru Z, Yining L. **Anti-tumor effect and protective effect on chemotherapeutic damage of water-soluble extracts from *Hedyotis diffusa*.** *Journal of Chinese Pharmaceutical Sciences.* 2002;11(2):54–57.
51. Xiaoming L, et al. **Effect of Yin Er, Fu Ling and Jiao Gu Lan on the immunological and free radical-clearing functions in mice.** *Journal of Beijing Medical University.* 1995;27(6):455–57,473.
52. Klein A, et al. **Pathway-focused bioassays and transcriptome analysis contribute to a better activity monitoring of complex herbal remedies.** *BMC Genomics.* February 27, 2013;14:133.
53. Liying L, et al. **Clinical observation on treating 40 cases of malignant ascites with intraperitoneal perfusion of Bai Hua She She Cao.** *Modern Tumour Medicine.* 2004;12(2):147.
54. Xiaoming L, et al. **Immune function restoring function and free radical clearing function of Jiao Gu Lan saponin and its compound in aged mice.** *Journal of Chinese Gerontics.* 1998;18(12):364–65.
55. Pacifico D, et al. **NMR-based metabolomics for organic farming traceability of early potatoes.** *J Agric Food Chem.* November 20, 2013;61(46):11201–11.
56. Gordon B. **Manganese nutrition of glyphosate-resistant and conventional soybeans.** *Better Crops.* 2007;91(4):12–13.
57. Hunter D, et al. **Evaluation of the micronutrient composition of plant foods produced by organic and conventional agricultural methods.** *Crit Rev Food Sci Nutr.* July 2011;51(6):571–82. Review.
58. Akbaba U, Sahin Y, Türkez H. **Element content analysis by WDXRF in pistachios grown under organic and conventional farming regimes for human nutrition and health.** *Toxicol Ind Health.* October 2012;28(9):783–88.
59. Vanzo A, et al. **Metabolomic profiling and sensorial quality of "Golden Delicious," "Liberty," "Santana," and "Topaz" apples grown using organic and integrated production systems.** *J Agric Food Chem.* July 3, 2013;61(26):6580–87.
60. Nitika PD, Khetarpaul N. **Physico-chemical characteristics, nutrient composition and consumer acceptability of wheat varieties grown under organic and inorganic farming conditions.** *Int J Food Sci Nutr.* May 2008;59(3):224–45.
61. Vallverdú-Queralt A, et al. **A metabolomic approach differentiates between conventional and organic ketchups.** *J Agric Food Chem.* November 9, 2011;59(21):11703–10.
62. Ruiz-Aracama A, et al. **Application of an untargeted metabolomics approach for the identification of compounds that may be responsible for observed differential effects in chickens fed an organic and a conventional diet.** *Food Addit Contam Part A Chem Anal Control Expo Risk Assess.* 2012;29(3):323–32.
63. Kazimierczak R, et al. **Beetroot (Beta vulgaris L.) and naturally fermented beetroot juices from organic and conventional production: Metabolomics, antioxidant levels and anticancer activity.** *J Sci Food Agric.* May 2, 2014.
64. Asami DK, et al. **Comparison of the total phenolic and ascorbic acid content of freeze-dried and air-dried marionberry, strawberry, and corn grown using conventional, organic, and sustainable agricultural practices.** *J Agric Food Chem.* 2003;51(5):1237–41.
65. Vrček IV, et al. **A comparison of the nutritional value and food safety of organically and conventionally produced wheat flours.** *Food Chem.* January 15, 2014;143:522–29.
66. Park YS, et al. **Nutritional and pharmaceutical properties of bioactive compounds in organic and conventional growing kiwifruit.** *Plant Foods Hum Nutr.* March 2013;68(1):57–64.
67. Palupi E, et al. **Comparison of nutritional quality between conventional and organic dairy products: a meta-analysis.** *J Sci Food Agric.* November 2012;92(14):2774–81. Review.
68. Hallmann E. **The influence of organic and conventional cultivation systems on the nutritional value and content of bioactive compounds in selected tomato types.** *J Sci Food Agric.* November 2012;92(14):2840–48.
69. Crinnion WJ. **Organic foods contain higher levels of certain nutrients, lower levels of pesticides, and may provide health benefits for the consumer.** *Altern Med Rev.* April 2010;15(1):4–12. Review.

Chapter 22: Mirror, Mirror

1. Abravanel ED. ***Dr. Abravanel's Body Type Diet and Lifetime Nutrition Plan.*** New York, NY: Bantam; 1999.

2. Cabot S, Cooper D, Burani JC. ***The Body-Shaping Diet.*** New York, NY: Warner Books; 1995.
3. Falchi M, et al. **Low copy number of the salivary amylase gene predisposes to obesity.** *Nat Genet.* May 2014;46(5):492–97.
4. Müller MJ, Bosy-Westphal A, Heymsfield SB. **Is there evidence for a set point that regulates human body weight?** *F1000 Med Rep.* August 9, 2010;2:59. doi:10.3410/M2-59.
5. Keesey RE, Corbett SW. **Metabolic defense of the body weight set-point.** *Res Publ Assoc Res Nerv Ment Dis.* 1984;62:87–96.
6. Pasquet P, Apfelbaum M. **Recovery of initial body weight and composition after long-term massive overfeeding in men.** *Am J Clin Nutr.* December 1994;60(6):861–63.
7. Speakman JR, et al. **Set points, settling points and some alternative models: theoretical options to understand how genes and environments combine to regulate body adiposity.** *Dis Model Mech.* November 2011;4(6):733–45.
8. Müller MJ, Bosy-Westphal A, Heymsfield SB. **Is there evidence for a set point that regulates human body weight?** *F1000 Med Rep.* August 9, 2010;2:59. doi: 10.3410/M2-59.
9. Keesey RE, Corbett SW. **Metabolic defense of the body weight set-point.** *Res Publ Assoc Res Nerv Ment Dis.* 1984;62:87–96.
10. Pasquet P, Apfelbaum M. **Recovery of initial body weight and composition after long-term massive overfeeding in men.** *Am J Clin Nutr.* December 1994;60(6):861–63.
11. Keesey RE, Corbett SW. **Metabolic defense of the body weight set-point.** *Res Publ Assoc Res Nerv Ment Dis.* 1984;62:87–96.
12. Brownell KD, et al. **The effects of repeated cycles of weight loss and regain in rats.** *Physiol Behav.* 1986;38(4):459–64.
13. Lim C-F, et al. **Transport of thyroxine into cultured hepatocytes: effects of mild nonthyroidal illness and calorie restriction in obese subjects.** *Clin Endocrinol* (Oxf). 1994;40:79–85.
14. Croxson MS, Ibbertson HK. **Low serum triiodothyronine (T3) and hypothyroidism in anorexia nervosa.** *J Clin Endorinol Metab.* 1977;44:167–74.
15. Manore MM, et al. **Energy expenditure at rest and during exercise in nonobese female cyclical dieters and in nondieting control subjects.** *Am J Clin Nutr.* 1991;54:41–46.
16. Lim C-F, et al. **A furan fatty acid and indoxyl sulfate are the putative inhibitors of thyroxine hepatocyte transport in uremia.** *J Clin Endocrinol Metab.* 1993;76:318–24.
17. Lim C-F, et al. **Inhibition of thyroxine transport into cultured rat hepatocytes by serum of non-uremic critically ill patients: effects of bilirubin and nonesterified fatty acids.** *J Clin Endocrinol Metab.* 1993;76:1165–72.
18. Brehm A, et al. **Increased lipid availability impairs insulin-stimulated ATP synthesis in human skeletal muscle.** *Diabetes.* 2006;55:136–40.
19. Tremblay A. **Dietary fat and body weight set point.** *Nutr Rev.* July 2004;62(7 Pt 2):S75–7. Review.
20. Cabanac M, Frankham P. **Evidence that transient nicotine lowers the body weight set point.** *Physiol Behav.* August 2002;76(4–5):539–42.
21. de Castro JM, Paullin SK, DeLugas GM. **Insulin and glucagon as determinants of body weight set point and microregulation in rats.** *J Comp Physiol Psychol.* June 1978;92(3):571–79.
22. Chaput JP, Tremblay A. **The glucostatic theory of appetite control and the risk of obesity and diabetes.** *Int J Obes* (Lond). January 2009;33(1):46–53. doi: 10.1038/ijo.2008.221.
23. Tappy L, Binnert C, Schneiter P. **Energy expenditure, physical activity and body-weight control.** *Proc Nutr Soc.* August 2003;62(3):663–66.
24. Meckling KA, Sherfey R. **A randomized trial of a hypocaloric high-protein diet, with and without exercise, on weight loss, fitness, and markers of the Metabolic Syndrome in overweight and obese women.** *Appl Physiol Nutr Metab.* August 2007;32(4):743–52.
25. Ibid.
26. Brehm BJ, D'Alessio DA. **Benefits of high-protein weight loss diets: enough evidence for practice?** *Curr Opin Endocrinol Diabetes Obes.* October 2008;15(5):416–21.
27. Stiegler P, Cunliffe A. **The role of diet and exercise for the maintenance of fat-free mass and resting metabolic rate during weight loss.** *Sports Med.* 2006;36(3):239–62.
28. Peters JC. **Dietary fat and body weight control.** *Lipids.* February 2003;38(2):123–27.
29. Gosselin C, Cabanac M. **Adrenalectomy lowers the body weight set-point in rats.** *Physiol Behav.* September 1997;62(3):519–23.
30. Farvid MS, et al. **Association of adiponectin and resistin with adipose tissue compartments, insulin resistance and dyslipidaemia.** *Diabetes, Obesity and Metabolism.* July 2005;7(4):406–13.
31. Ross R, et al. **Adipose tissue volume measured by magnetic resonance imaging and computerized tomography in**

rats. *J Appl Physiol.* May 1, 1991;70:2164–72.

32. Urbanchek MG, et al. **Specific force deficit in skeletal muscles of old rats is partially explained by the existence of denervated muscle fibers.** *Journals of Gerontology Series A: Biological Sciences and Medical Sciences.* May 1, 2001;56(5):B191–B197.
33. Elia M. **Organ and tissue contribution to metabolic weight.** In: Kinney JM, Tucker HN, eds. ***Energy Metabolism: Tissue Determinants and Cellular Corollaries.*** New York, NY: Raven Press; 1999: 61–79.
34. Donnelly JE, et al. **Is resistance training effective for weight management?** *Evidence-Based Preventive Medicine.* 2003;1(1):21–29.
35. Srikanthan P, Hevener AL, Karlamangla AS. **Sarcopenia exacerbates obesity-associated insulin resistance and dysglycemia: findings from the national health and nutrition examination survey III.** *PLoS One.* May 26, 2010;5(5):e10805.
36. Rhéaume C, et al. **Contributions of cardiorespiratory fitness and visceral adiposity to six-year changes in cardiometabolic risk markers in apparently healthy men and women.** May 1, 2011;96(5):1462–68.
37. Hutchison SK, et al. **Effects of exercise on insulin resistance and body composition in overweight and obese women with and without polycystic ovary syndrome.** *J Clin Endocrinol Metab,* January 1, 2011;96(1):E48–E56.
38. Srikanthan P, Karlamangla AS. **Relative muscle mass is inversely associated with insulin resistance and prediabetes. Findings from the third National Health and Nutrition Examination Survey.** *J Clin Endocrinol Metab.* September 2011;96(9)2898–903.
39. Evans WJ, Campbell WW. **Sarcopenia and age-related changes in body composition and functional capacity.** *J Nutr.* February 1993;123(2 Suppl):465–68.
40. Morley JE. **Anorexia, sarcopenia, and aging.** *Nutr.* July–August 2001;17(7–8):660–63.
41. Ford ES, Maynard LM, Li C. **Trends in mean waist circumference and abdominal obesity among US adults, 1999–2012.** *JAMA.* 2014;312(11):1151–53.
42. Briggs DI, et al. **Calorie-restricted weight loss reverses high-fat diet-induced ghrelin resistance, which contributes to rebound weight gain in a ghrelin-dependent manner.** *Endocrinology.* February 2013;154(2):709–17.
43. Lustig RH. **The neuroendocrinology of obesity.** *Endocrinol Metab Clin North Am.* September 2001;30(3):765–85.
44. McNay DE, Speakman JR. **High fat diet causes rebound weight gain.** *Mol Metab.* November 2012;2(2):103–108.

Chapter 23: Secrets to Weight Loss?

1. Hill AJ. **Does dieting make you fat?** *British Journal of Nutrition.* August 2004;92(S1):S15–S18.
2. Ibid.
3. Elia M. **Organ and tissue contribution to metabolic weight.** In: Kinney JM, Tucker HN, eds. ***Energy Metabolism: Tissue Determinants and Cellular Corollaries.*** New York, NY: Raven Press; 1992: 61–79.
4. Ibid.
5. Ibid.
6. Levine JA, et al. **Interindividual variation in posture allocation: possible role in human obesity.** *Science.* January 2005;307(5709):584–86.
7. Ibid.
8. Hill AJ. **Does dieting make you fat?** *British Journal of Nutrition.* August 2004;92(S1):S15–S18.
9. Elia M. **Organ and tissue contribution to metabolic weight.** In: Kinney JM, Tucker HN, eds. ***Energy Metabolism: Tissue Determinants and Cellular Corollaries.*** New York, NY: Raven Press; 1992: 61–79.
10. Meerman R, Brown AJ. **When somebody loses weight, where does the fat go?** *BMJ.* 2014;349.
11. Ibid.
12. Keim NL, Barbieri TF, Van Loan M. **Physiological and biochemical variables associated with body fat loss in overweight women.** *Int J Obes.* April 1991;15(4):283–93.
13. Poirier P, Després JP. **Exercise in weight management of obesity.** *Cardiol Clin.* August 2001;19(3):459–70.
14. Rosenkilde M, et al. **Body fat loss and compensatory mechanisms in response to different doses of aerobic exercise—a randomized controlled trial in overweight sedentary males.** *Am J Physiol Regul Integr Comp Physiol.* September 15, 2012;303(6):R571–R579.
15. Smith TJ, et al. **Efficacy of a meal-replacement program for promoting blood lipid changes and weight and body fat loss in US Army soldiers.** *J Am Diet Assoc.* February 2010;110(2):268–73.

16. Willis FB, Smith FM, Willis AP. **Frequency of exercise for body fat loss: a controlled, cohort study.** *J Strength Cond Res.* November 2009;23(8):2377–80.
17. Krebs JD, et al. **Changes in risk factors for cardiovascular disease with body fat loss in obese women.** *Diabetes Obes Metab.* November 2002;4(6):379–87.
18. Lamarche B, et al. **Is body fat loss a determinant factor in the improvement of carbohydrate and lipid metabolism following aerobic exercise training in obese women?** *Metabolism.* November 1992;41(11):1249–56.
19. Tremblay A, Nadeau A, Bouchard C. **Is body fat loss a determinant factor in the improvement of carbohydrate and lipid metabolism following aerobic exercise training in obese women?** *Metabolism.* November 1992;41(11):1249–56.
20. Ballor DL, Poehlman ET. **Exercise-training enhances fat-free mass preservation during diet-induced weight loss: a meta-analytical finding.** *Int J Obes Relat Metab Disord.* January 1994;18(1):35–40.
21. Donnelly JE, et al. **Is resistance training effective for weight management?** *Evidence-Based Preventive Medicine.* 2003;1:21–29.
22. Farnsworth E, et al. **Effect of a high-protein, energy-restricted diet on body composition, glycemic control, and lipid concentrations in overweight and obese hyperinsulinemic men and women.** *Am J Clin Nutr.* July 2003;78(1):31–39.
23. Katch FI, Michael ED Jr., Jones EM. **Effects of physical training on the body composition and diet of females.** American Association for Health, Physical Education and Recreation. *Research Quarterly.* 1969;40(1):99–104.
24. Muth DM. **What are the guidelines for percentage of body fat loss?** ACE Fitness. December 2, 2009. https://www.acefitness.org/acefit/healthy-living-article/60/112/what-are-the-guidelines-for-percentage-of/.
25. Troisi RJ, et al. **Relation of obesity and diet to sympathetic nervous system activity.** *Hypertension.* 1991;17:669–77.
26. Gibala MJ, et al. **Physiological adaptations to low-volume, high-intensity interval training in health and disease.** *J Physiol.* March 1, 2012;590(Pt 5):1077–84.
27. Gibala MJ, McGee SL. **Metabolic adaptations to short-term high-intensity interval training: A little pain for a lot of gain?** *Exerc Sport Sci Rev.* April 2008;36(2):58–63.
28. Little JP, Francois ME. **High-intensity interval training for improving postprandial hyperglycemia.** *Res Q Exerc Sport.* December 2014;85(4):451–56.
29. Álvarez C, et al. **Eight weeks of combined high intensity intermittent exercise normalized altered metabolic parameters in women.** *Rev Med Chil.* April 2014;142(4):458–66.
30. Ho SS, Dhaliwal SS, Hills AP, Pal S. **The effect of 12 weeks of aerobic, resistance or combination exercise training on cardiovascular risk factors in the overweight and obese in a randomized trial.** *BMC Public Health.* August 28, 2012;12:704.
31. De Feo P. **Is high-intensity exercise better than moderate-intensity exercise for weight loss?** *Nutr Metab Cardiovasc Dis.* November 2013;23(11):1037–42.
32. Ballor DL, Poehlman ET. **Exercise-training enhances fat-free mass preservation during diet-induced weight loss: a meta-analytical finding.** *Int J Obes Relat Metab Disord.* January 1994;18(1):35–40.
33. Farnsworth E, et al. **Effect of a high-protein, energy-restricted diet on body composition, glycemic control, and lipid concentrations in overweight and obese hyperinsulinemic men and women.** *Am J Clin Nutr.* July 2003;78(1):31–39.
34. Katch FI, Michael ED Jr., Jones EM. **Effects of physical training on the body composition and diet of females.** American Association for Health, Physical Education and Recreation. *Research Quarterly.* 1969;40(1):99–104.
35. Ibid.
36. Muth DM. **What are the guidelines for percentage of body fat loss?** ACE Fitness. December 2, 2009. https://www.acefitness.org/acefit/healthy-living-article/60/112/what-are-the-guidelines-for-percentage-of/.
37. Pasiakos SM, et al. **Effects of high-protein diets on fat-free mass and muscle protein synthesis following weight loss: a randomized controlled trial.** *FASEB J.* September 2013;27(9):3837–47.
38. Soenen S, et al. **Normal protein intake is required for body weight loss and weight maintenance, and elevated protein intake for additional preservation of resting energy expenditure and fat free mass.** *J Nutr.* May 2013;143(5):591–96.
39. Gibala MJ, et al. **Physiological adaptations to low-volume, high-intensity interval training in health and disease.** *J Physiol.* March 1, 2012;590(Pt 5):1077–84.
40. Abbas A, Szczepaniak LS, Tuncel M, et al. **Adiposity-independent sympathetic activity in black men.** *Journal of Applied Physiology.* June 1, 2010;108:1613–18.
41. Grassi G, et al. **Body weight reduction, sympathetic nerve traffic, and arterial baroreflex in obese normotensive**

humans. *Circulation*. 1998;15(97):2037–42.

42. Grassi G, Seravelle G, Cattaneo BM, et al. **Sympathetic activation in obese normotensive subjects**. *Hypertension*. 1995;25:560–63.
43. Gudbjornsdottir S, et al. **Sympathetic nerve activity and insulin in obese normotensive and hypertensive men**. *Hypertension*. February 1996;27(2):276–80.
44. Scherrer U, et al. **Body fat and sympathetic nerve activity in healthy subjects**. *Circulation*. 1994;89(6):2634–40.
45. National Institute of Child Health and Human Development staff. **Stress system malfunction could lead to serious, life threatening disease.** NICHD/NIH. July 21, 2006. http://www.nichd.nih.gov/news/releases/pages/stress.aspx.
46. Bakris G, et al. **Atlas vertebra realignment and achievement of arterial pressure goal in hypertensive patients: a pilot study**. *J Human Hyperten*. May 2007;21(5):347–52.
47. Edwards IJ, Deuchars SA, Deuchars J. **The intermedius nucleus of the medulla: a potential site for the integration of cervical information and the generation of autonomic responses**. *J Clin Neuroanatomy*. November 2009;38(3)166–75.
48. Matteoli G, Boeckxstaens GE. **The vagal innervation of the gut and immune homeostasis**. *Gut*. August 2013;62(8):1214–22.
49. Welch A, Boone R. **Sympathetic and parasympathetic responses to specific diversified adjustments to chiropractic vertebral subluxations of the cervical and thoracic spine**. *J Chiropractic Medicine*. September 2008;7(3):86–93.
50. Nance DM, Sanders VM. **Autonomic innervation and regulation of the immune system**. *Brain Behav Immun*. August 2007;21(6):736–45.
51. Jowsey P, Perry J. **Sympathetic nervous system effects in the hands following a grade III postero-anterior rotatory mobilisation technique applied to T4: a randomized, placebo-controlled trial**. *Man Ther*. June 2010;15(3):248–53.
52. Pickar JG. **Neurophysiological effects of spinal manipulation**. *Spine Journal*. September–October 2002;2(5):357–71.
53. Sterling M, Jull G, Wright A. **Cervical mobilisation: concurrent effects on pain, sympathetic nervous system activity and motor activity**. *Man Ther*. May 2011;6(2):72–81.
54. Budgell B, Polus B. **The effects of thoracic manipulation on heart rate variability: a controlled crossover trial**. *Journal of Manipulative and Physiological Therapeutics*. October 2006;29(8):603–61.
55. Gibbons PF, Gosling CM, Holmes M. **Short-term effects of cervical manipulation on edge light pupil cycle time: A pilot study.** *Journal of Manipulative and Physiological Therapeutics*. September 2000;23(7):465–69.39.
56. Banni S, et al. **Vagus nerve stimulation reduces body weight and fat mass in rats**. *PloS One*. September 28, 2012.
57. McClelland J, et al. **A systematic review of the effects of neuromodulation on eating and body weight: evidence from human and animal studies**. *Eur Eat Disorders Rev*. November 2013;21:436–55.
58. Rubin R, Nazario B. **The skinny on next generation weight loss treatments.** *Medscape Diabetes & Endocrinology*. March 2, 2015.
59. Uddén J, et al. **Effects of glucocorticoids on leptin levels and eating behaviour in women.** *J Intern Med*. February 2003;253(2):225–31.
60. Farvid MS, et al. **Association of adiponectin and resistin with adipose tissue compartments, insulin resistance and dyslipidaemia.** *Diabetes, Obesity and Metabolism*. July 2005;7(4):406–13.
61. Landsberg L. **Hyperinsulinemia: Possible role in obesity-induced hypertension**. *Hypertension*. January 1992;19(1 Suppl):161–66.
62. Holmberg I, et al. **Absorption of a pharmacological dose of vitamin D3 from two different lipid vehicles in man: comparison of peanut oil and a medium chain triglyceride.** *Biopharm Drug Dispos*. December 1990;11(9):807–15.
63. De Ridder CM, et al. **Body fat mass, body fat distribution, and plasma hormones in early puberty in females.** *J Clin Endocrinol Metab*. April 1, 1990;70(4):888–93.
64. Miller M. **Mayo Clinic study on low estrogen and weight gain unclear.** Healthline. May 10, 2013. http://www.healthline.com/health-blogs/hold-that-pause/mayo-clinic-study-low-estrogen-weight-gain-unclear.
65. Cumming DC, Quigley ME, Yen SS. **Acute suppression of circulating testosterone levels by cortisol in men.** *J Clin Endocrinol Metab*. September 1983;57(3):671–73.
66. Ibid.
67. Bambino TH, Hsueh AJ. **Direct inhibitory effect of glucocorticoids upon testicular lutenizing hormone receptor and steroidogenesis in vivo and in vitro.** *Endocrinology*. June 1981;108(2):2142–48.
68. Brownlee KK, et al. **Relationship between circulating cortisol and testosterone: influence of physical exercise.** *Journal of Sports Science and Medicine*. March 2005;4:76–83.

69. McClelland J, et al. **A systematic review of the effects of neuromodulation on eating and body weight: evidence from human and animal studies.** *Eur Eat Disorders Rev*. November 2013;21:436–55.
70. Miller M. **Mayo Clinic study on low estrogen and weight gain unclear.** *Healthline*. May 10, 2013. http://www.healthline.com/health-blogs/hold-that-pause/mayo-clinic-study-low-estrogen-weight-gain-unclear.
71. Uddén J, et al. **Effects of glucocorticoids on leptin levels and eating behaviour in women.** *J Intern Med*. February 2003;253(2):225–31.
72. Masuzaki H, et al. **Transgenic amplification of glucocorticoid action in adipose tissue causes high blood pressure in mice.** *J Clin Invest*. July 2003;112(1):83–90.
73. Ibid.
74. Bambino TH, Hsueh AJ. **Direct inhibitory effect of glucocorticoids upon testicular lutenizing hormone receptor and steroidogenesis in vivo and in vitro.** *Endocrinology*. June 1981;108(2):2142–48.
75. Varughese AG, Nimkevych O, Uwaifo GI. **Hypercortisolism in obesity-associated hypertension.** *Curr Hypertens Rep*. July 2014;16(7):443.
76. De Leo M, et al. **Subclinical Cushing's syndrome.** *Best Pract Res Clin Endocrinol Metab*. August 2012;26(4):497–505.

Chapter 24: Fat Children? Act Now!

1. Salans LB, Cushman SW, Weismann RE. **Studies of human adipose tissue. Adipose cell size and number in nonobese and obese patients.** *J Clin Invest*. April 1973;52(4):929–41.
2. **Childhood obesity facts.** Centers for Disease Control. February 27, 2014. http://www.cdc.gov/healthyyouth/obesity/facts.htm.
3. Ibid.
4. Wang S. **Fatty liver disease: more prevalent in children.** *Wall Street Journal*. Updated September 9, 2013. http://online.wsj.com/news/articles/SB10001424127887324549004579064903051692782.
5. Spalding KL, et al. **Dynamics of fat cell turnover in humans.** *Nature*. June 5, 2008;453:783–87.
6 Ibid.
7. Salans LB, Cushman SW, Weismann RE. **Studies of human adipose tissue. Adipose cell size and number in nonobese and obese patients.** *J Clin Invest*. April 1973;52(4):929–41.
8. Spalding KL, et al. **Dynamics of fat cell turnover in humans.** *Nature*. June 5, 2008;453:783–87.
9. Cunningham S, Kramer M, Narayan V. **Incidence of childhood obesity in the United States.** *N Engl J Med*. January 30, 2014;370:403–11.
10. Kolata G. **Obesity is found to gain its hold in earliest years.** *New York Times*. January 29, 2014. http://www.nytimes.com/2014/01/30/science/obesity-takes-hold-early-in-life-study-finds.html?module=Search&mabReward=relbias percent3Ar&_r=0.
11. Ibid.
12. Cunningham S, Kramer M, Narayan V. **Incidence of childhood obesity in the United States.** *N Engl J Med*. January 30, 2014;370:403–11.
13. de Assis S, et al. **High-fat or ethinyl-oestradiol intake during pregnancy increases mammary cancer risk in several generations of offspring.** *Nat. Commun*. September 11, 2012;3:1053.
14. Martinez-Chacin RC, Keniry M, Dearth RK. **Analysis of high fat diet induced genes during mammary gland development: Identifying role players in poor prognosis of breast cancer.** *BMC Res Notes*. August 18, 2014;7(1):543.
15. Montales MT, et al. **Maternal metabolic perturbations elicited by high-fat diet promote Wnt-1-induced mammary tumor risk in adult female offspring via long-term effects on mammary and systemic phenotypes.** *Carcinogenesis*. September 2014;35(9):2102–112.
16. Vogt MC, et al. **Neonatal insulin action impairs hypothalamic neurocircuit formation in response to maternal high fat feeding.** *Cell*. January 30, 2014;156(3)495–509.
17. Montales MT, et al. **Maternal metabolic perturbations elicited by high-fat diet promote Wnt-1-induced mammary tumor risk in adult female offspring via long-term effects on mammary and systemic phenotypes.** *Carcinogenesis*. September 2014;35(9):2102–112.
18. Vogt MC, et al. **Neonatal insulin action impairs hypothalamic neurocircuit formation in response to maternal high fat feeding.** *Cell*. January 30, 2014;156(3)495–509.
19. Ibid.

20. Mina TH, Reynolds RM. **Mechanism linking in utero stress to altered offspring behaviour.** *Curr Top Behav Neurosci.* February 28, 2014. (Epub ahead of print.)
21. Weinstock M. **The long-term consequences of stress on brain function: from adaptations to mental diseases.** *Neuroscience & Biobehavioral Reviews.* August 2008;32(6):1073–86.
22. Lester BM, Conradt E, Marsit CJ. **Fetal origins of adult disease: epigenetic basis for the development of depression in children.** *Clin Obstet & Gynocol.* September 2013;56(3):556–65.
23. Mina TH, Reynolds RM. **Mechanism linking in utero stress to altered offspring behaviour.** *Curr Top Behav Neurosci.* February 28, 2014. (Epub ahead of print.)
24. Lester BM, Conradt E, Marsit CJ. **Fetal origins of adult disease: epigenetic basis for the development of depression in children.** *Clin Obstet & Gynocol.* September 2013;56(3):556–65.
25. Raine A, et al. **Reduction in behavior problems with omega-3 supplementation in children aged 8–16 years: a randomized, double-blind, placebo-controlled, stratified, parallel-group trial.** *Journal of Child Psychology and Psychiatry.* 2015;56(5):509.
26. Rhee KE, McEachern R, Jelalian E. **Parent readiness to change differs for overweight child dietary and physical activity behaviors.** *Journal of the Academy of Nutrition and Dietetics.* June 20, 2014.
27. Lundahl A, Kidwell KM, Nelson TD. **Parental underestimates of child weight: A meta-analysis.** *Pediatrics.* March 1, 2014;133(3):e689–e703.
28. Rhee KE, McEachern R, Jelalian E. **Parent readiness to change differs for overweight child dietary and physical activity behaviors.** *Journal of the Academy of Nutrition and Dietetics.* June 20, 2014.
29. Epstein LH, et al. **Randomized trial of the effects of reducing television viewing and computer use on body mass index in young children.** *Arch Pediatr Adolesc Med.* March 2008;162(3):239–45.
30. Vigdor J, Ladd, H. **Scaling the Digital Divide: Home Computer Technology and Student Achievement.** Urban Institute. August 10, 2010. http://www.urban.org/research/publication/scaling-digital-divide-home-computer-technology-and-student-achievement.
31. Khandaker GM, et al. **Association of serum interleukin 6 and C-reactive protein in childhood with depression and psychosis in young adult life: A population-based longitudinal study.** *JAMA Psychiatry.* 2014;71(10):1121–28.
32. Ibid.
33. Wang X, et al. **Inflammatory markers and risk of type 2 diabetes: a systematic review and meta-analysis.** *Diabetes Care.* January 2013;36(1):166–75.
34. Suglia SF, Kara S, Robinson WR. **Sleep duration and obesity among adolescents transitioning to adulthood: Do results differ by sex?** *Journal of Pediatrics.* 2014.
35. Condezo-Hoyos L, Mohanty IP, Noratto GD. **Assessing non-digestible compounds in apple cultivars and their potential as modulators of obese faecal microbiota in vitro.** *Food Chemistry.* 2014;161:208.
36. Chudnovskiy R, et al. **Consumption of clarified grapefruit juice ameliorates high-fat diet induced insulin resistance and weight gain in mice.** *PLoS One.* 2014;9(10):e108408.

Chapter 25: When Health Goes Up, Weight Goes . . .

1. World Health Organization. **Obesity: Preventing and Managing the Global Epidemic: Report of a WHO Consultation (WHO Technical Report Series 894).** Geneva, Switzerland: World Health Organization; 2000: 39.
2. Ekelund U, et al. **Physical activity and all-cause mortality across levels of overall and abdominal adiposity in European men and women: The European Prospective Investigation into Cancer and Nutrition Study (EPIC).** *Am J Clin Nutr.* January 14, 2015.
3. Brüning JC, et al. **Role of brain insulin receptor in control of body weight and reproduction.** *Science.* September 22, 2000;289(5487):2122–25.
4. Hunt KF, Cheah YS, Amiel SA. **Brain insulin resistance.** In: Byrne CD and Wild SH: ***The Metabolic Syndrome.*** Sussex, UK: Wiley-Blackwell; 2011: 139–64.
5. Cheatham RA, et al. **Long-term effects of provided low and high glycemic load low energy diets on mood and cognition.** *Physiol Behav.* September 7, 2009;98(3):374–79.
6. Hanley AJ, et al. **Elevations in markers of liver injury and risk of type 2 diabetes: The insulin resistance atherosclerosis study.** *Diabetes.* October 2004;53(10):2623–32.
7. Kelley DE, et al. **Fatty liver in type 2 diabetes mellitus: relation to regional adiposity, fatty acids, and insulin resistance.**

Am J Physiol Endocrinol Metab. October 2003;285(4):E906–E916.

8. Ryysy L, et al. **Hepatic fat content and insulin action on free fatty acids and glucose metabolism rather than insulin absorption are associated with insulin requirements during insulin therapy in type 2 diabetic patients.** *Diabetes*. May 2000;49(5):749–58.
9. Seppälä-Lindroos A, et al. **Fat accumulation in the liver is associated with defects in insulin suppression of glucose production and serum fatty acids independent of obesity in normal men.** *J Clin Endocrinol Metab*. July 2002;87(7):3023–28.

Chapter 26: Eating Chocolate to Lose Weight!

1. Kwok CS, et al. **Habitual chocolate consumption and risk of cardiovascular disease among healthy men and women.** *Heart*. June 15, 2015.
2. Tierney J. **Do you suffer from decision fatigue?** *New York Times Magazine*. August 21, 2011.
3. Baumeister RF. **The Psychology of Irrationality.** In Brocas I and Carrillo JD, *The Psychology of Economic Decisions: Rationality and Well-Being*. Oxford, UK: Oxford University Press; 2003: 1–15.
4. Danziera S, Levav J, Avnaim-Pesso L. **Extraneous factors in judicial decisions.** *Proceedings of the National Academy of Sciences*. 2011;108(17):6889–92.
5. Brooks SJ, et al. **A debate on current eating disorder diagnoses in light of neurobiological findings: Is it time for a spectrum model?** *BMC Psychiatry*. 2012;12(76).
6. Baeken C, Claes S, De Raedt R. **The influence of COMT ValMet genotype on the character dimension cooperativeness in healthy females.** *Brain and Behavior*. 2014,4:515–20.
7. Schroeder JA, et al. **Nucleus accumbens C-Fos expression is correlated with conditioned place preference to cocaine, morphine and high fat/sugar food consumption.** Neuroscience Conference, 2013; Annual Meetings/Neuroscience 2013 Abstracts. (Unpublished.)
8. Pelletier C, et al. **Associations between weight loss-induced changes in plasma organochlorine concentrations, serum T(3) concentration, and resting metabolic rate.** *Toxicol Sci*. May 2002;67(1):46–51.
9. Ibid.
10. Ibid.
11. Ziegler TR, et al. **Increased intestinal permeability associated with infection in burn patients.** *Arch Surg*. 1988;123(11):1313–19.
12. Ledingham JG, et al. **Effects of aging on vasopressin secretion, water excretion, and thirst in man.** *Kidney Int Suppl*. August 1987;21:S90–S92.
13. Stachenfeld NS, et al. **Mechanism of attenuated thirst in aging: role of central volume receptors.** *Am J Physiol*. January 1997;272(1 Pt 2):R148–R157.
14. Rolls BJ, Phillips PA. **Aging and disturbances of thirst and fluid balance.** *Nutr Rev*. March 1990;48(3):137–44. Review.
15. Farrell MJ, et al. **Effect of aging on regional cerebral blood flow responses associated with osmotic thirst and its satiation by water drinking: A PET study.** *Proc Natl Acad Sci USA*. January 8, 2008;105(1):382–87.
16. Kenney WL, Chiu P. **Influence of age on thirst and fluid intake.** *Med Sci Sports Exerc*. September 2001;33(9):1524–32. Review.
17. Vij VA, Joshi AS. **Effect of "water induced thermogenesis" on body weight, body mass index and body composition of overweight subjects.** *J Clin Diagn Res*. September 2013;7(9):1894–96.
18. Davy BM, et al. **Water consumption reduces energy intake at a breakfast meal in obese older adults.** *J Am Diet Assoc*. July 2008;108(7):1236.
19. Batmanghelidi F. ***Your Body's Many Cries for Water.*** Vienna, VA: Global Health Solutions; 2008.
20. Smith JL. Review: **The role of gastric acid in preventing foodborne disease and how bacteria overcome acid conditions.** *J Food Prot*. July 2003;66(7):1292–303. Review.
21. Karamanolis G, et al. **A glass of water immediately increases gastric pH in healthy subjects.** *Dig Dis Sci*. 2008.
22. Tennant SM, et al. **Bacterial infections: Influence of gastric acid on susceptibility to infection with ingested bacterial pathogens.** *Infect Immun*. February 2008;76(2):639–45.
23. Morihara M, et al. **Assessment of gastric acidity of Japanese subjects over the last 15 years.** *Biol Pharm Bull*. March 2001;24(3):313–15.

Chapter 27: Just Chew It!

1. Malamud D, et al. **Antiviral activities in human saliva.** *Adv Dent Res.* April 2011;23(1):34–37. Review.
2. Luo H, et al. **Isolation, purification and antibacterial activities of salivary histidine-rich polypeptides.** *Hua Xi Kou Qiang Yi Xue Za Zhi (West China Journal of Stomatology).* August 1999;17(3):227–29, 232. Chinese.
3. Lange J. **Some humoral factors in human saliva having antiinfectious activities due to chemical properties.** *Tandlaegebladet.* October 1967;71(10):918–31. Danish.
4. Nauntofte B, Jensen JL. **Salivary secretion.** In: Yamada T, et al., eds. ***Textbook of Gastroenterology***, 3rd ed. Philadelphia, PA: Lippencott Williams, Wilkins Publishers; 1999: 263–78.
5. Pedersen A, et al. **Saliva and gastrointestinal functions of taste, mastication, swallowing and digestion.** *Oral Diseases.* 2002;8:117–29.
6. Pacific Health Laboratories. **A calorie is not a calorie.** Training Peaks. December 20, 2012. http://home.trainingpeaks.com/blog/article/a-calorie-is-not-a-calorie.
7. Burmeister MA, et al. **Central glucagon-like peptide 1 receptor-induced anorexia requires glucose metabolism-mediated suppression of AMPK and is impaired by central fructose.** *Am J Physiol Endocrinol Metab.* April 1 2013;304(7):E677–E685.
8. Yadav H, et al. **Epigenomic derangement of hepatic glucose metabolism by feeding of high fructose diet and its prevention by Rosiglitazone in rats.** *Dig Liver Dis.* July 2009;41(7):500–8.
9. Maiztegui B, et al. **Islet adaptive changes to fructose-induced insulin resistance: beta-cell mass, glucokinase, glucose metabolism, and insulin secretion.** *J Endocrinol.* February 2009;200(2):139–49.
10. Teff KL, et al. **Endocrine and metabolic effects of consuming fructose- and glucose-sweetened beverages with meals in obese men and women: influence of insulin resistance on plasma triglyceride responses.** *J Clin Endocrinol Metab.* May 2009;94(5):1562–69.
11. Daly ME, et al. **Dietary carbohydrates and insulin sensitivity: A review of the evidence and clinical implications.** *Am J Clin Nutr.* 1997;66:1072–85.
12. Hollenbeck CB. **Dietary fructose effects on lipoprotein metabolism and risk for coronary artery disease.** *Am J Clin Nutr.* November 1993;58(5 Suppl):800S–809S.
13. Kallus SJ, Brandt LJ. **The intestinal microbiota and obesity.** *J Clin Gastroenterol.* 2012 Jan;46(1):16–24.
14. Krych Ł, et al. **Gut microbial markers are associated with diabetes onset, regulatory imbalance, and IFN-γ level in NOD Mice.** *Gut Microbes.* February 2015;3:0.
15. Kiecolt-Glaser JK, et al. **Daily stressors, past depression, and metabolic responses to high-fat meals: a novel path to obesity.** *Biological Psychiatry.* 2014.
16. Zeevi D, et al. **Personalized Nutrition by Prediction of Glycemic Responses.** *Cell.* November 1990; 63(5):1079–94.
17. Le Chatelier E, et al. **Richness of human gut microbiome correlates with metabolic markers.** *Nature.* August 29, 2013;500(7464:541–46.
18. Carpenter D, et al. **Obesity, starch digestion and amylase: association between copy number variants at human salivary (AMY1) and pancreatic (AMY2) amylase genes.** *Hum Mol Genet.* June 15, 2015;24(12):3472–80.
19. Dunstan DW, et al. **Breaking up prolonged sitting reduces postprandial glucose and insulin responses.** *Diabetes Care.* May 2012;35(5):976–83. doi: 10.2337/dc11-1931. Epub February 28, 2012.
20. Himsworth HP. **Dietetic factors influencing glucose tolerance and the activity of insulin.** *J Physiol.* March 29, 1934;81(1):29–48.
21. Nago N, et al. **Low cholesterol is associated with mortality from stroke, heart disease, and cancer: The Jichi Medical School Cohort Study.** *J Epidemiol.* 2011;21(1):67–74.
22. Simko V, Ginter E. **Understanding cholesterol: High is bad but too low may also be risky—is low cholesterol associated with cancer?** *Bratisl Lek Listy.* 2014;115(2):59–65.
23. Koton S, et al. **Low cholesterol, statins and outcomes in patients with first-ever acute ischemic stroke.** *Cerebrovasc Dis.* 2012;34(3):213–20.
24. Chung YH, et al. **Statins of high versus low cholesterol-lowering efficacy and the development of severe renal failure.** *Pharmacoepidemiol Drug Saf.* June 2013;22(6):583–92.
25. Ginter E, Kajaba I, Sauša M. **Addition of statins into the public water supply? Risks of side effects and low cholesterol levels.** *Cas Lek Cesk.* 2012;151(5):243–47.

26. Zhang J. **Epidemiological link between low cholesterol and suicidality: a puzzle never finished.** *Nutr Neurosci.* November 2011;14(6):268–87.
27. Frost G, et al. **The short-chain fatty acid acetate reduces appetite via a central homeostatic mechanism.** *Nature Communications.* May 2014.
28. Behall KM, Howe JC. **Resistant starch as energy.** *J Am Coll Nutr.* June 1996;15(3):248–54.
29. Cummings H, Macfarlane GT, Englyst HN. **Prebiotic digestion and fermentation.** *Am J Clin Nutr.* 2001;73(2 Suppl):415S–420S.
30. Phillips J, et al. **Effect of resistant starch on fecal bulk and fermentation-dependent events in humans.** *American Journal of Clinical Nutrition.* July 1995;62(1):121–30.
31. Greer JB, O'Keefe SJ. **Microbial induction of immunity, inflammation, and cancer.** *Front Physiol.* 2011;1:168.
32. Johnston KL, et al. **Resistant starch improves insulin sensitivity in metabolic syndrome.** *Diabetic Medicine.* 2010;27:391–97.
33. Gorissen SH, et al. **Carbohydrate coingestion delays dietary protein digestion and absorption but does not modulate postprandial muscle protein accretion.** *J Clin Endocrinol Metab.* June 2014;99(6):2250–58.
34. Watson WC, Paton E. **Studies on intestinal pH by radiotelemetering.** *Gut.* 1965;6:606–12.
35. Fallingborg J. **Intraluminal pH of the human gastrointestinal tract.** *Dan Med Bull.* June 1999;46(3):183–96. Review.
36. Evans DF, et al. **Measurement of gastrointestinal pH profiles in normal ambulant human subjects.** *Gut.* August 1988;29(8):1035–41.
37. Beck IT. **The role of pancreatic enzymes in digestion.** *Am J Clin Nutr.* 1973;26:311–25.
38. Dangin M, et al. **The rate of protein digestion affects protein gain differently during aging in humans.** *J Physiology.* June 1, 2003;549:635–44.
39. Barnosky AR, et al. **Intermittent fasting vs. daily calorie restriction for type 2 diabetes prevention: A review of human findings.** *Transl Res.* June 12, 2014.
40. Manzanero S, et al. **Intermittent fasting attenuates increases in neurogenesis after ischemia and reperfusion and improves recovery.** *J Cereb Blood Flow Metab.* May 2014;34(5):897–905.
41. Vasconcelos AR, et al. **Intermittent fasting attenuates lipopolysaccharide-induced neuroinflammation and memory impairment.** *J Neuroinflammation.* May 6, 2014;11:85.
42. Azevedo FR, Ikeoka D, Caramelli B. **Effects of intermittent fasting on metabolism in men.** *Rev Assoc Med Bras.* March–April 2013;59(2):167–73.
43. Kahleová H, et al. **Eating two larger meals a day (breakfast and lunch) is more effective than six smaller meals in a reduced-energy regimen for patients with type 2 diabetes: a randomised crossover study.** *Diabetologia.* May 2014.
44. Steen S, Oppliger RA, Brownell KD. **Metabolic effects of repeated weight loss and regain in adolescent wrestlers.** *JAMA.* July 1,1988;260(1):47–50.
45. Isaacson W. ***Einstein: His Life and Universe.*** New York, NY: Simon & Schuster; 2008.
46. Dunstan DW, et al. **Breaking up prolonged sitting reduces postprandial glucose and insulin responses.** *Diabetes Care.* May 2012;35(5):976–83. doi: 10.2337/dc11-1931. Epub February 28, 2012.

Chapter 28: Gonna Keep Pumping Air in That Tire?

1. Hicks LA, Taylor TH, Hunkler RJ. **U.S. outpatient antibiotic prescribing, 2010.** *N Engl J Med.* April 11, 2013;368:1461–62.
2. Caverly TJ, et al. **Too much medicine happens too often: the teachable moment and a call for manuscripts from clinical trainees.** *JAMA Intern Med.* 2014;174(1):8–9.

Chapter 29: On Healing and Rainbows

1. Choi SW, Friso S. **Epigenetics: A new bridge between nutrition and health.** *Adv Nutr.* November 2010;1:8–16.
2. Vickers MH. **Developmental programming and adult obesity: The role of leptin.** *Curr Opin Endocrinol Diabetes Obes.* February 2007;14(1):17–22.
3. Waterland RA, et al. **Methyl donor supplementation prevents transgenerational amplification of obesity.** *International Journal of Obesity.* September 2008;32(9):1373–79.
4. Soubry A, et al. **Newborns of obese parents have altered DNA methylation patterns at imprinted genes.** *Int J Obes.* October 25, 2013.
5. Dubovsky S. **Emerging Perspectives: Epigenetics—a mechanism for the impact of experience on inheritance?** *NEJM*

Journal Watch. October 18, 2010. http://www.jwatch.org/jp201010180000001/2010/10/18/emerging-perspectives-epigenetics-mechanism.

6. Khalyfa A, et al. **Effects of late gestational high-fat diet on body weight, metabolic regulation and adipokine expression in offspring.** *Int J Obes (Lond).* November 2013;37(11):1481–89.
7. Haig D. **The (dual) origin of epigenetics.** Cold Spring Harbor Symposia on Quantitative Biology. Cold Spring Harbor, NY. June 6, 2004. http://www.oeb.harvard.edu/faculty/haig/Publications_files/04EpigeneticOrigins.pdf.
8. Painter RC, Roseboom TJ, Bleker OP. **Prenatal exposure to the Dutch famine and disease in later life: An overview.** *Reprod Toxicol.* September 2005;20(3):345–52.
9. Heijmans BT, et al. **Persistent epigenetic differences associated with prenatal exposure to famine in humans.** *Proc Natl Acad Sci USA.* November 4, 2008;105(44):17046–49.
10. Soubry A, et al. **Paternal obesity is associated with IGF2 hypomethylation in newborns: Results from a Newborn Epigenetics Study (NEST) cohort.** *BMC Med.* 2013;11:29.
11. Bianconi E, et al. **An estimation of the number of cells in the human body.** *Ann Hum Biol.* November–December 2013;40(6):463–71.

Chapter 31: The Essential You: Deeper Meanings to Illness

1. Sanford JA. ***Healing and Wholeness.*** Mahwah, NJ: Paulist Press; 1997.
2. Jung C. ***Memories, Dreams, Reflections.*** New York, NY: Pantheon Press; 1961.

Chapter 32: Help for Deep Healing: Life's Toolbox

1. de Almeida AA, et al. **Differential effects of exercise intensities in hippocampal BDNF, inflammatory cytokines and cell proliferation in rats during the postnatal brain development.** *Neurosci Lett.* October 11, 2013; 553:1–6.
2. Tuon T, et al. **Physical training prevents depressive symptoms and a decrease in brain-derived neurotrophic factor in Parkinson's disease.** *Brain Res Bull.* September 28, 2014; 108C:106–12.
3. Berretta A, Tzeng YC, Clarkson AN. **Post-stroke recovery: The role of activity-dependent release of brain-derived neurotrophic factor.** *Expert Rev Neurother.* November 2014;14(11):1335–44.
4. **Transcendental meditation: What is the TM technique?** Transcendental Meditation. 2014. http://www.tm.org/.
5. **Miracles in your life.** Video. Eckankar. Updated June 4, 2014. http://www.eckankar.org/Video/play.php?name=Miracles+in+Your+Life.
6. Bhargava R, Gogate MG, Mascarenhas JF. **Autonomic responses to breath holding and its variations following pranayama.** *Indian J Physiol Pharmacol.* 1988;42:257–64.
7. Sakakibara M, Hayano J. **Effect of slowed respiration on cardiac parasympathetic response to threat.** *Psychosom Med.* 1996;58:32–37.
8. Telles S, Nagarathna R, Nagendra HR. **Breathing through a particular nostril can alter metabolism and autonomic activities.** *Indian J Physiol Pharmacol.* 1994;38:133–37.
9. Mohan M, et al. **Effect of yoga type breathing on heart rate and cardiac axis of normal subjects.** *Indian J Physiol Pharmacol.* 1986;30:334–40.
10. Khanam AA, et al. **Study of pulmonary and autonomic functions of asthma patients after yoga training.** *Indian J Physiol Pharmacol.* 1996;40:318–24.
11. Alabdulgader AA. **Coherence: A Novel Nonpharmacological Modality for Lowering Blood Pressure in Hypertensive Patients.** *Global Advances in Health and Medicine.* May 2012;1(2):54–62.
12. Sanford JA. ***Healing and Wholeness.*** Mahwah, NJ: Paulist Press; 1997.
13. Pergameni CG. Hatzopoulos O, ed. ***That the Best Physician Is Also a Philosopher, with a Modern Greek Translation.*** Athens, Greece: Odysseas Hatzopoulos & Co.: Kaktos Editions; 1992.
14. Oberhelman SM. **Galen, on diagnosis from dreams.** *J Hist Med Allied Sci.* January 1983;38(1):36–47.

Chapter 34: The Reason Why

1. Jung C. ***Memories, Dreams, Reflections.*** New York, NY: Pantheon Press; 1961.
2. Klemp H. ***The Art of Spiritual Dreaming.*** Chanhassen, MN: Eckankar; 1999.
3. Sanford JA. ***Dreams: God's Forgotten Language.*** Philadelphia, PA: J. B. Lippincott; 1968.

Index

About the Author

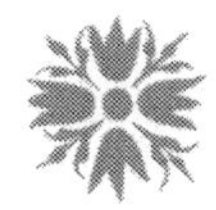

Dr. Luis Arrondo is a cum laude graduate of Parker University of Chiropractic. He has worked with Stanford Medical University's Family Medicine Core Clerkship Program to help Stanford medical students learn more about alternative healing approaches when they visit his clinic. He developed his expansive, multidisciplinary view of health and the body's innate ability to heal while traveling and practicing in the United States and Italy. He is certified in Neurochemistry and Nutrition from the American College of Functional Neurology, has served as a State Certified Qualified Medical Examiner and as a Fellow of the Academy of Forensic and Industrial Chiropractic Consultants, and has been certified in the Neuro Emotional Technique. He has lived in five countries and now practices in San Jose, California. He enjoys bicycling and discovering more about the connections between our health and our physical, mental, and spiritual dynamics.

Made in the USA
Lexington, KY
19 June 2018